THE WAY OF
ENERGY

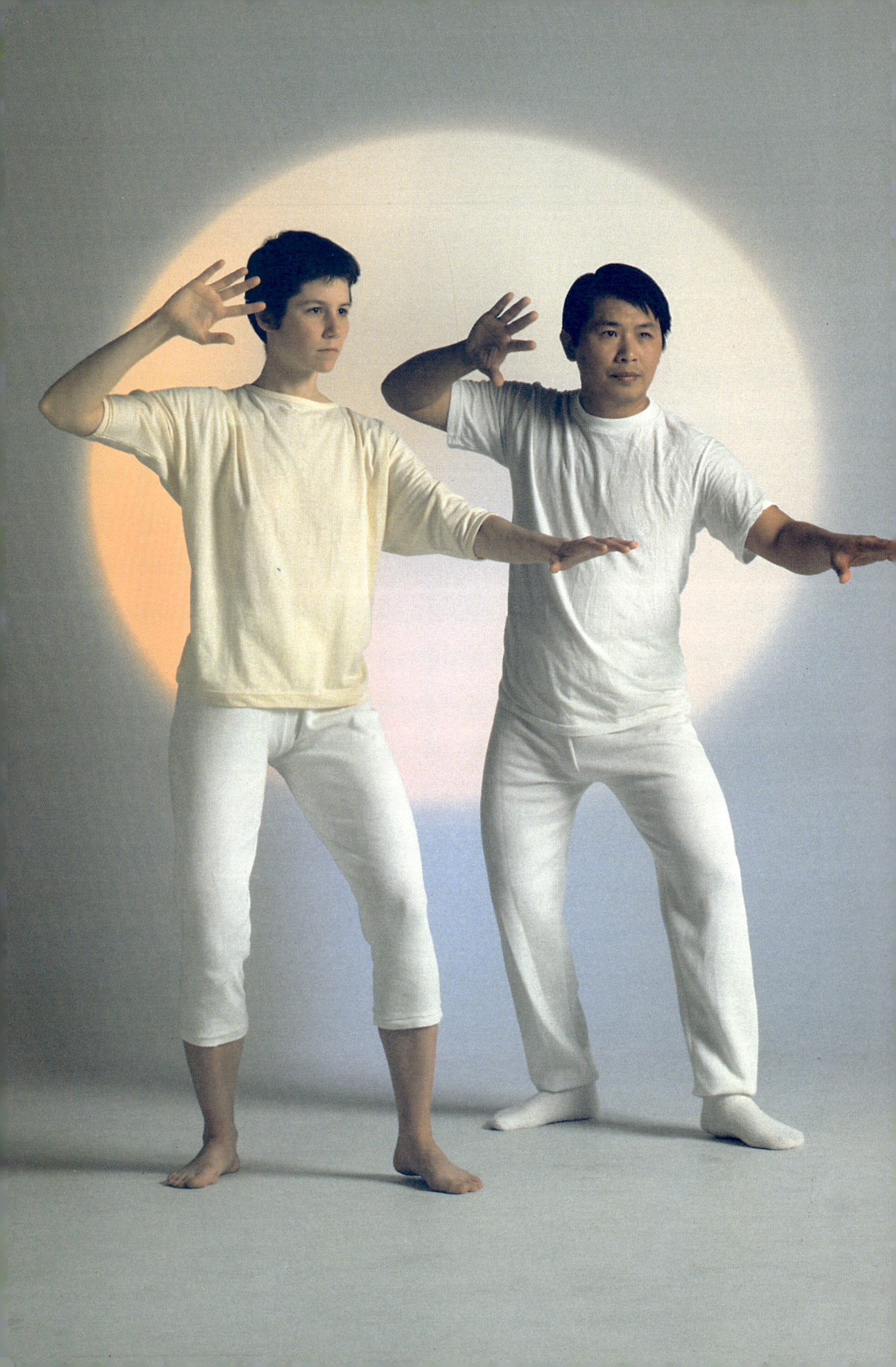

THE WAY OF ENERGY

Mastering the Art of Internal Strength with Chi Kung Exercise

Master Lam Kam Chuen

Gaia Books Limited

A GAIA ORIGINAL

Editorial Eleanor Lines
Katherine Pate

Design Gail Langley

Photography Fausto Dorelli

Illustration Paul Beebee

Direction Joss Pearson
Patrick Nugent

First published in the United Kingdom in 1991 by
Gaia Books Limited *and*
66 Charlotte Street 20 High Street, Stroud
London W1P 1LR Gloucestershire GL5 1AS

Typeset by Tradespools Ltd, Somerset, UK
Reproduction by Fotographics Ltd, Hong Kong
Printed and bound in Spain by Mateu Cromo

British Library Cataloguing in Publication Data
Chuen, Lam Kam
Way of energy
1. Humans. Alternative therapy
615.5

ISBN 1-85675-020-5

10 9 8 7 6

CAUTION
The techniques, ideas, and suggestions in this book are not intended as a substitute for proper medical advice. Any application of the techniques, ideas and suggestions in this book is at the reader's sole discretion and risk.

How to Use this Book

This book will help you master the basic Zhan Zhuang system of Chi Kung internal energy exercise. The instructions are based on the experience of many masters and their students: if you follow them precisely you will be in safe hands.

Part One introduces the warm ups and the first two standing exercises and outlines the sensations that you may feel when beginning or progressing to a new level. Part Two takes you on to the intermediate level, with a more powerful series of warm up exercises, and three more standing positions. The four most advanced postures are introduced in Part Three, along with "mentality exercises", which are visualization techniques used to enhance the effectiveness of the postures. Part Four explains how Zhan Zhuang can be incorporated into everyday life. The last chapter deals with the self-treatment of minor ailments.

The techniques presented in this book are available to people of all ages and levels of fitness. Chapter 9 gives programmes for those starting Zhan Zhuang at different stages of life, for example, in middle age, and for the elderly. It is very important to respect the advice on each of the exercises and not to skip ahead to try out something that is too advanced for you.

Unlike keep-fit systems that set fixed regimes, Zhan Zhuang allows for your individuality. You can progress at your own pace, working carefully and systematically through the exercises, following the guidelines in Parts One to Three of this book. Once you are comfortable doing each exercise, you will be able to create a daily programme of your own, drawing on the postures and techniques you have learned.

Like all good exercise systems, regular practice is essential. There is no point in rushing ahead, seeking instant results. Zhan Zhuang works on your internal energy patterns and usually manifests external results only after a few months. If you practise these exercises as part of your daily routine, you will continue to develop your internal power over a whole lifetime.

The drawings and photographs in this book have been supervised by Master Lam Kam Chuen. If you are able to find a qualified instructor, this book will be a permanent resource for your training.

A WORD OF CAUTION

Positions 6 to 9 (pp. 104–119) in this book have a strong effect on your circulatory system and, as with all intense exercise, push up your blood pressure during the period of training. Attempt these positions only if your doctor advises that your normal blood pressure level will permit this.

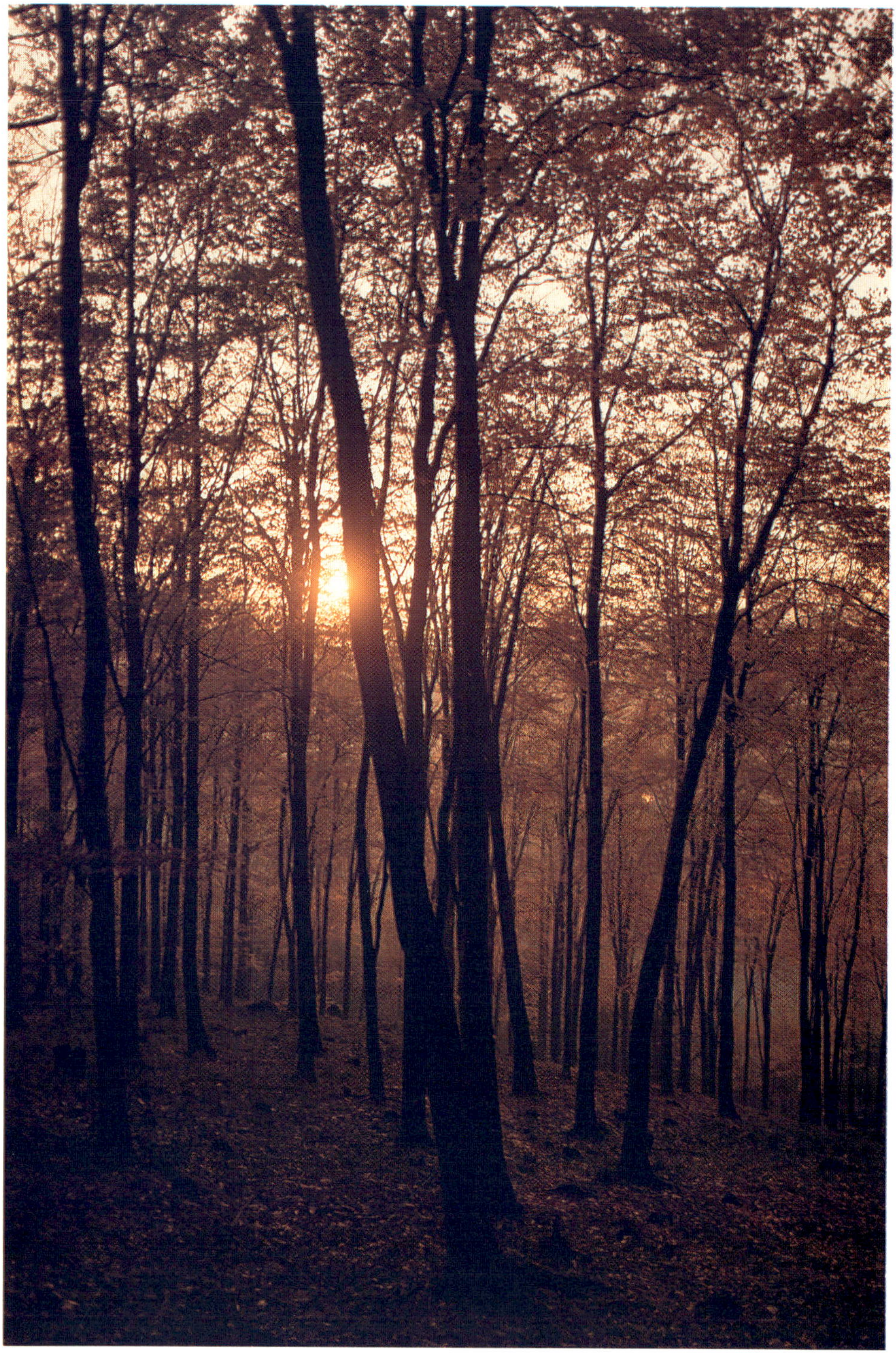

Contents

How to Use this Book 5

Foreword 8
Introduction 11

Part One 23
Chapter 1 Learning to Stand 25
Chapter 2 Breathing and Relaxing 41
Chapter 3 Internal Movement 51

Part Two 61
Chapter 4 Preparing for Energy 63
Chapter 5 Growing Like a Tree 83

Part Three 101
Chapter 6 Roots and Branches 103
Chapter 7 Going Beyond 123

Part Four 139
Chapter 8 Energy in Daily Life 141
Chapter 9 The Life Cycle 159
Chapter 10 Taking Care of Yourself 173

Index 189
Acknowledgements, Resources,
and Bibliography 191

FOREWORD

by
Professor Yu Yong Nian
Honorary Member of the Council of the Association of Chi Kung Science of the People's Republic of China and adviser to the American – Chinese Chi Kung Association.

For centuries the art of internal strength was a closely guarded secret in China. Embracing all the hard and soft martial arts including Tai Chi and Chi Kung, it is only now that it is being unveiled, both in my country and to the world outside.

My experience of the extraordinary benefits of the Zhan Zhuang style of Chi Kung exercise stretches over the past 50 years, during which time I have studied its application in hospitals and clinics throughout China. People of all ages have come to be treated for disorders that often neither Western medicine nor traditional Chinese medicine could cure: hypertension; arthritis; some tumours, and other chronic disorders of the respiratory, cardiovascular, and nervous systems.

The time has come to make this system of preventative and therapeutic health care open to everyone. *The Way of Energy* makes a unique contribution to understanding the health and potential that is the natural heritage of every human being. I am pleased to have been able to collaborate in this with Master Lam Kam Chuen of Hong Kong. A qualified practitioner of traditional Chinese medicine, he has contributed to my own experience as a surgeon in the Western medical tradition, both through his own research in the ancient study of Chi (vital energy) and through his years of clinical work healing people with bone, nerve, and muscle injuries.

It is rare to find an authentic master of an ancient art. Since the age of 12, Lam Kam Chuen has devoted himself to the internal strengthening and healing of the human body. Since those early days he has studied under masters in Hong Kong, Taiwan, and China, embracing a traditional range of studies that includes herbal medicine, the martial arts, the great religious philosophies of Chinese culture, and classical Chinese opera. He is one of the most highly trained and deeply knowledgeable experts in the art of healing and the study of internal strength currently practising and teaching in the Western world. Master Lam is the founder of the first and only clinic of its type in Europe for treating people on the basis of this powerful yet profoundly natural system. The clinic, opened in 1991, can be found near the heart of London's Chinatown.

Master Lam invited one of his students, Richard Reoch, to work with him in creating *The Way of Energy*, the first reference book on Zhan Zhuang for the Western reader. Born into a Buddhist family in Canada in 1948, Richard Reoch is one of a small group of people who began studying Zhan Zhuang under Master Lam in the 1980s. Working together for more than a year, and drawing on Master Lam's own knowledge, his library of Chinese texts, his Western medical works, and the experience of his students and patients, they have distilled a whole culture and a completely different way of understanding human beings into a form penetrable by the Western mind.

This book is a great achievement and I am delighted to think that *The Way of Energy* will be read in many countries and languages all over the world. I trust that everyone who has the opportunity to study it will be rewarded by its immense, hidden treasure.

Yu Yong Nian
November 1990

于永年
一九九〇年十一月

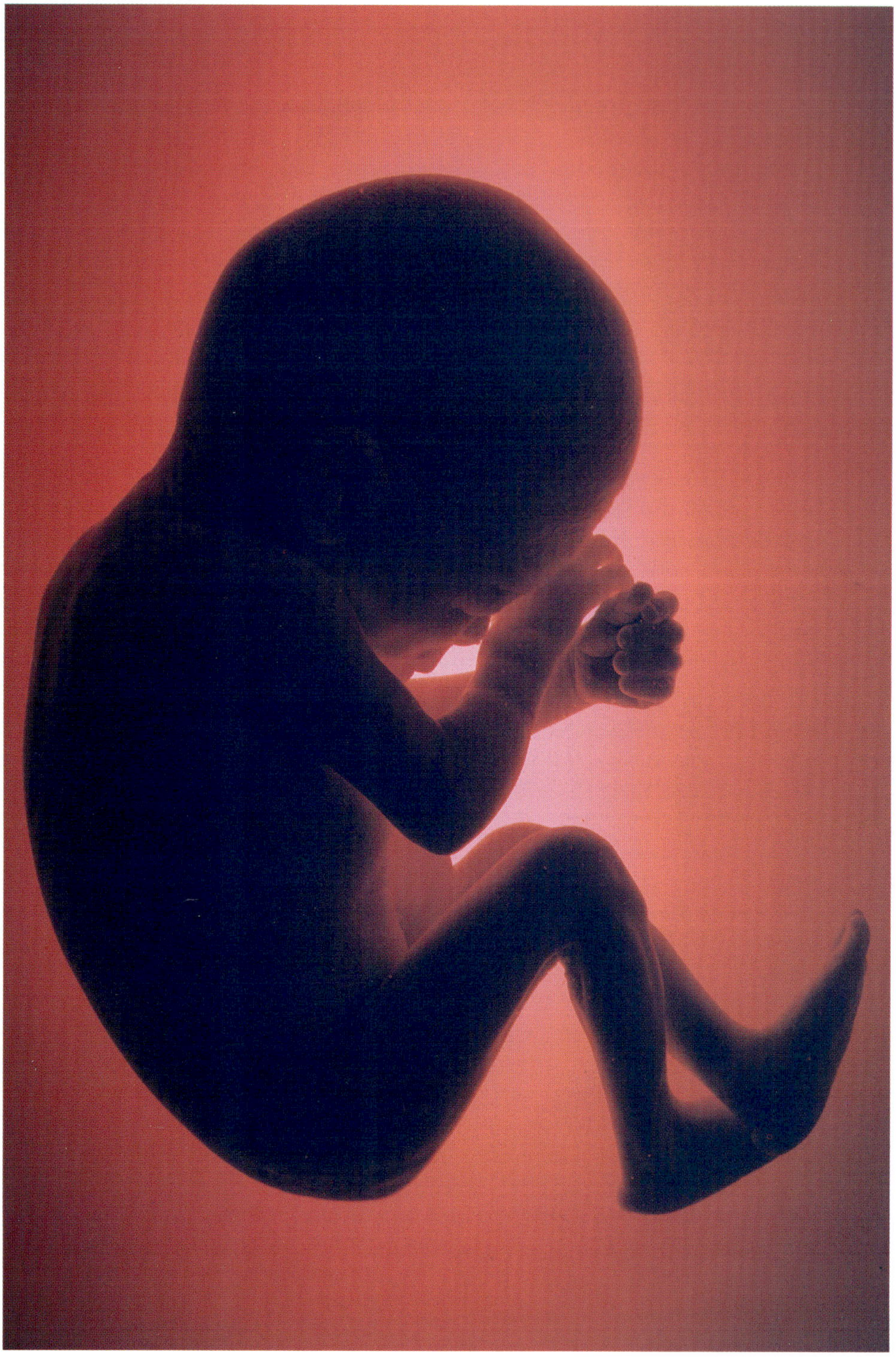

INTRODUCTION

In the early morning, before the hubbub of daily life, Chinese people of all ages begin the day by performing traditional exercises in the parks and woods wherever they live. You will see some doing rhythmic stretching movements – others are training in the martial arts. A common sight is Tai Chi Chuan, the exquisite slow exercise, one of the soft martial arts, that develops and relaxes the whole body. The first time that you see so many people, some in their eighties and others in their very early youth, all peacefully training together under the trees, is one of life's unforgettable moments.

But as you look more closely you may come across an even more remarkable sight. Among all these moving forms, here and there you will see some figures that rivet your attention. They are like the trees themselves. They are fully alive, but they are utterly still.

Although there is no obvious movement, they are deeply engaged in one of the most demanding and powerful forms of exercise ever developed. It is so utterly focused on deep, internal growth that it literally requires learning to stand like a tree. It is known in Chinese as Zhan Zhuang, "standing like a stake", or "standing like a tree". It is pronounced "Jan Jong", or, in southern China, "Jam Jong". This is the system to which you are about to be introduced in this book.

Like a tree with its deep roots, powerful trunk, and great spreading branches reaching into the sky, you will appear to remain unmoving. In reality you will be growing from within. Previously shrouded in secrecy, this health system is now attracting considerable international attention and scientific examination. The results are unmistakable: strengthened immunity; successful treatment of chronic illness; high levels of daily energy and the natural regeneration of the nervous system.

The Zhan Zhuang system of energy exercises takes most people completely by surprise, because although it is most definitely an energetic system of exercise, it involves virtually no movement! Unlike almost all other exercise methods, which consume energy, this actually generates energy. How is this possible? The answer lies in the nature of energy in the human body: how it is produced, and how it moves within the body.

YOUR NATURAL ENERGY

Our bodies are filled with energy, but it is blocked within us. We are born bursting with life, yet we grow old depleted of vitality.

Zhan Zhuang is a unique exercise that reverses this process of decay. Developed in China, it builds up and releases an extraordinary flow of natural energy that is dormant inside us, and raises the body and mind to remarkably high levels of fitness.

The energy in our bodies is so natural and so spontaneous, we almost never stop to think about it. It is like the constant rhythm of our lungs and the ceaseless circulation of our blood. Thousands upon thousands of chemical reactions are taking place at any one moment and countless electrical impulses are passing through every part of the system. Not only that, but we are all part of the entire flow of energy around us. The intricate networks of energy in your body form part of the energy of the natural world. You are a miniature field of the electromagnetic energy of the universe.

ORIGINS OF ENERGY

We begin with the fusion of the life energies of our parents. From the moment of conception, a new pattern of vitality is born and begins to grow. Floating effortlessly in the fluid of the womb, we absorb nutrition, protection, and immunity. We move with the rhythm of our mothers' bodies. Sustenance flows into us through the umbilical cord at the centre of our emerging being.

But from the moment of birth we undergo radical changes. The sustenance that previously came to us in the womb must now come from elsewhere. We are forced to draw it in for ourselves using our lungs, mouths, senses, and muscles.

Over time, even the way we breathe begins to change. At first we breathe naturally, from the belly, as if still centred around the umbilical cord. But as we age, the centre of breathing gradually moves upward in the torso, so that by late childhood most people think that they control their breathing with their chest muscles. Little by little, just staying alive causes tension to accumulate in our chests, shoulders, necks, and brains.

From the moment we first open our eyes as newborn babies our lives fill up with motion. We see everything around us constantly moving. Our bodies are continuously experiencing nervous and muscular tension of one sort or another. Our minds are endlessly being pulled this way or that. Even when we sleep,

"ARE THEY CHEATING ME?"

The first time someone told me to stand like a tree I didn't believe them. I was in my early twenties at the time. I had grown up in Hong Kong and trained to be a traditional Chinese doctor. Since I was 12 I had studied martial arts and been to many tournaments. By most people's standards you would have to say I was a serious martial artist and was physically fit. Now here was someone telling me: "If you want to learn the real thing, you should stand still without moving." It looked like nothing, but I tried it. I couldn't believe it: whatever was going on, it was far more demanding than any of the countless hours of hard physical exercise I had put in during my youth.

For several years after that I tried to find a competent Zhan Zhuang teacher. When I succeeded, I was told only one thing: stand without moving. I asked many questions but got no reply. I was told: "Just do it". For one year that was all I was taught. I began to ask myself: "Am I stupid? Are they cheating me?" But I continued practising every day and after one year when my teacher saw that I was prepared to stand like that and not ask questions, he started to explain it to me!

Slowly I began to understand what was happening inside my body. I started to know my own internal power. My whole approach changed, including my approach to the martial arts. Then, because I was continuing my traditional medical practice, I was told I ought to contact Professor Yu Yong Nian, a dentist and master of Zhan Zhuang in Beijing, who, in turn, had studied under Wang Xiang Zhai, the Grandmaster of Zhan Zhuang in its modern form. After a long correspondence, we finally met and eventually I was able to train under him and learn not only the exercise system but also its powerful application in the healing arts.

These days, even after all the years of training and study, I understand exactly what my students must be thinking at the very beginning when I show them how to stand and then tell them: "Just do it!". I think to myself: years ago I didn't believe any of this. It seems to defy everything we have been brought up to think. But I know it is the real thing. I just hope more people will be patient enough to realize it!

research has shown that our mental activity continues. If you ask people to stop thinking for a few moments and just forget everything, you will most likely find that they simply cannot do it. Their minds continue to scamper around like a monkey.

The mental tensions in our lives have a direct and disastrous effect on everything else. A very high proportion of the most common ailments that afflict people are related to tension – either as a direct result of it, such as headaches, heart attacks, and nervous disorders, or indirectly, as a result of the body's internal organs and immune system being weakened by tension in the muscles, organs, and nerves.

We rarely relax. Our original state of tranquil growth is lost to us. We move about in the air, but we are unable to rest in it as we once were able to rest in the waters of the womb. People try all sorts of ways to relax: watching television; listening to music; jogging; eating and, of course, sleeping. Others find yoga and meditation helpful. But only rarely do any of these ways relax both the nervous system and the entire muscle system.

In the practice of Zhan Zhuang, however, we can find a way to relax the nervous and the muscular systems simultaneously. This clears the pathway for the renewed circulation of the original, natural energy in our bodies and minds.

Doing this is the secret of the Way of Energy.

CULTIVATING INTERNAL STRENGTH

Using your original natural energy does not mean entering into a weak, mindless trance. Relaxing does not mean going limp. The secret of the art of internal strength is to rediscover and release the powerful energy that is dormant and blocked within you.

Complete relaxation is only one part of the process; the other is the development of mental and physical capacities that have lain untapped since birth. It is common knowledge that we use only a tiny percentage of our brain cells. It is also true that we are aware of and train only a percentage of our physical capacity. Most forms of exercise – running, swimming, weight training, team sports, and aerobics classes – concentrate on developing our physical strength. Most develop key muscle groups and have a powerful effect on the lungs, heart, and cardiovascular system. But there is a limit to the extent and benefit of such exercise. Long before your muscles are worked to their full capacity, the demand on your heart and particularly on your lungs is so

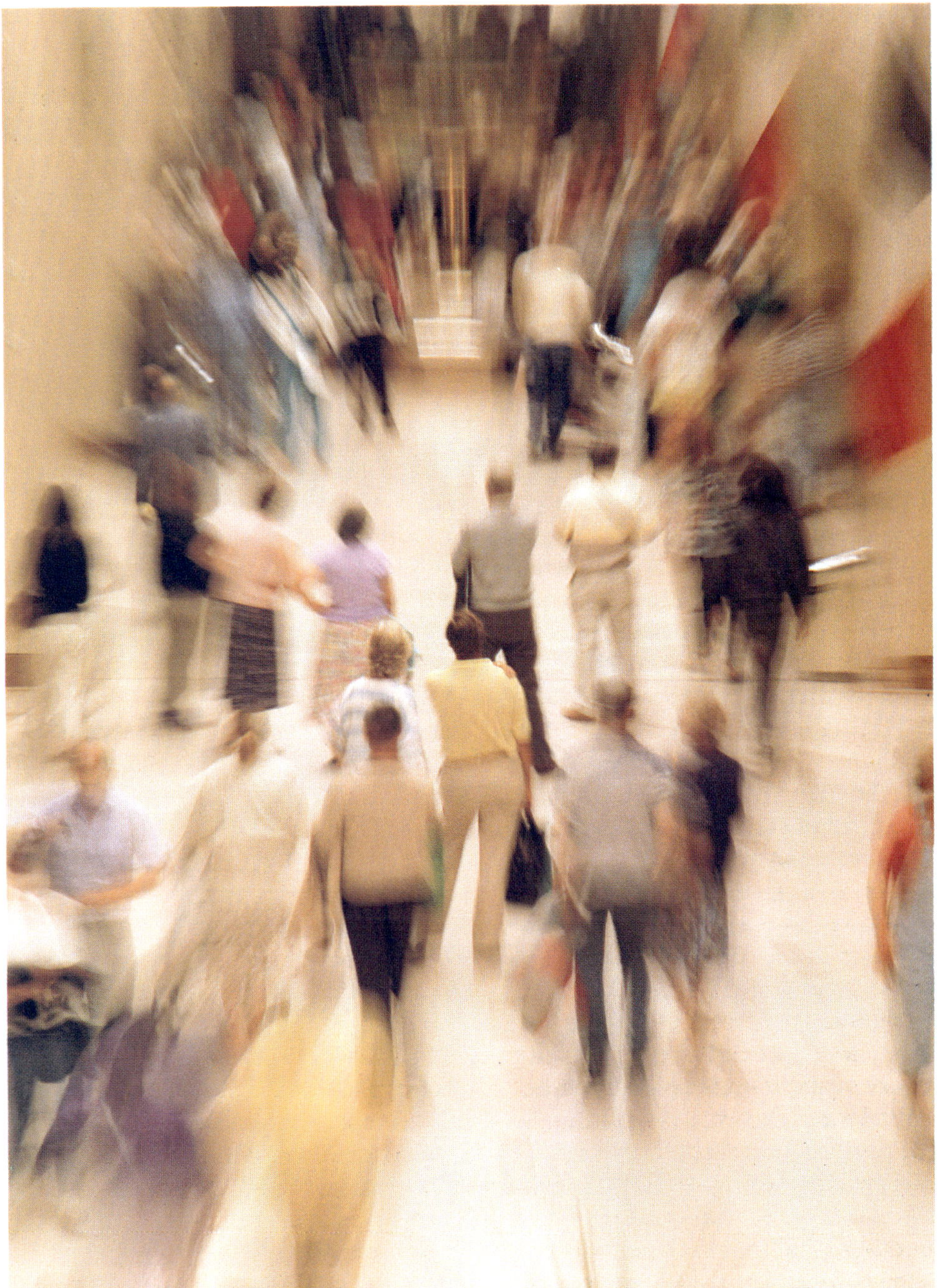

intense that sooner or later you become fatigued and must stop. The result is not only temporary exhaustion, but limited development of your muscle power.

The Zhan Zhuang exercises outlined in this book will enable you to exert the full capacity of your muscle networks over long periods without exhausting your lungs. In fact, your breathing will become even deeper and slower, generating a generous supply of oxygen to your heart. At the same time, your pulse rate will rise, enabling your heart to carry these high volumes of oxygen to your muscles and internal organs. Even though you will be exercising yourself as never before, you will not be left gasping grotesquely for air. You will be able to exercise without fighting against yourself. Very few other forms of exercise stimulate, cleanse, and massage all the body's internal systems in this way.

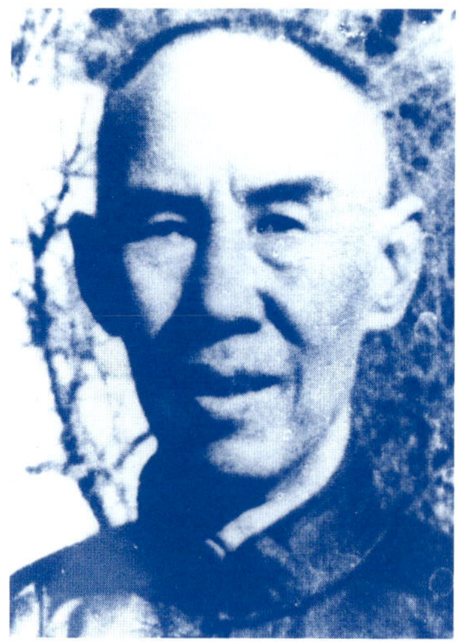

Wang Xiang Zhai

EXERTION AND RELAXATION

To accomplish this total cleansing and strengthening and to reduce radically the level of muscular and nervous tension in your body at the same time requires a completely different approach to exercise. It requires a method of training that combines exertion and relaxation simultaneously. This is different from doing vigorous exercise, such as calisthenics, and following this with a resting period. The Way of Energy is based on a dynamic and simultaneous fusion of exertion and relaxation – two apparently contradictory activities.

For people unfamiliar with the fundamentals of traditional Chinese medicine, the results of this system of exercise may seem to border on the magical, and those who believe in them may seem to border on the gullible! But as interest in alternative medicine gathers momentum and people begin to think about health and fitness in new and challenging ways, there is now a fresh willingness to look more deeply into the wisdom and experience that has been handed down to us from other centuries and other cultures.

YOU ARE LIKE THE HIBERNATING DRAGON

In the mid-1940s an announcement appeared in the Chinese newspaper Shibao *and in some other journals outside China inviting anyone to come and beat up a middle-aged gentleman living in Beijing! No one who took up the challenge ever succeeded. No wonder – they had tried to overcome Wang Xiang Zhai, the founder of a form of martial art known as Great Achievements Shadow Boxing, or Da Cheng Chuan.*

The basic training for anyone who wishes to practise Da Cheng Chuan (pronounced Da-chen-chwan) is the series of standing exercises of Zhan Zhuang. As Master Wang himself explained to his students, "Action originates in inaction and stillness is the mother of movement."

Master Wang's style was the result of years of study. As a child he suffered from poor health and was encouraged to improve his physical condition by taking up martial arts training under Master Guo Yunshan who lived in his village.

After Master Guo's death, Wang Xiang Zhai spent the next 10 years travelling throughout China meeting and studying under the great martial arts masters of the day.

By the mid-1940s, Wang Xiang Zhai was ready to launch his new style, Da Cheng Chuan, and came to Beijing where he was soon recognized as a master of extraordinary wisdom and prowess.

To help his students, who spent hours under his guidance, standing like a tree, Master Wang composed verses that condensed the essence of his teaching:

"Propelled by natural strength,
You are as strong as a dragon.
Inhaling and exhaling naturally and quietly,
You perceive the mechanism of all movement.

Avail yourself of the force of the Universe,
And bring your instinctive ability into full play.

In motion you are like the angry tiger,
In quietness you are like the hibernating dragon."

THE CHINESE WAY

The Chinese have studied the energy of the human body for thousands of years. This study is one of the earliest activities recorded in human civilization and dates back to the reign of the Yellow Emperor (thought to have been 2690-2590 BC). It continues to expand and develop to this very day. The results form a sophisticated and meticulous body of knowledge bringing together three disciplines usually treated as completely separate in the West: medicine, philosophy, and the martial arts.

Central to the Chinese analysis of energy and its behaviour is the concept of Chi (pronounced "chee"). The Chinese character for Chi (see above) has several meanings. It can mean "air" or "breath", but it is most commonly used to represent the concept of

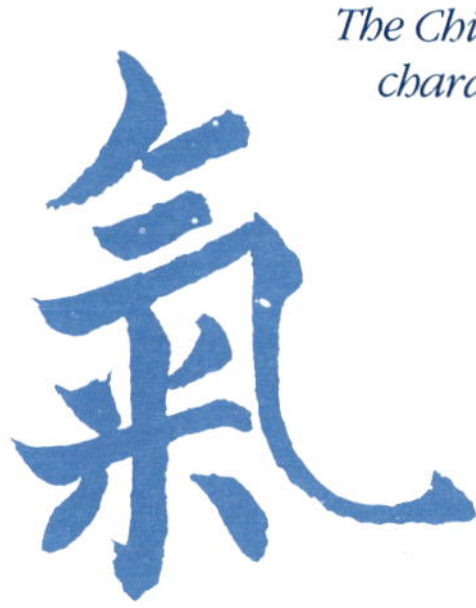

The Chinese character Chi.

"energy" or "vital essence". In the human body, Chi is the fundamental energy that sustains life and is present in the vibrating biological processes of every single one of the millions and millions of cells. It drives all the activities throughout the organism. This energy is not uniquely human. Every being shares in and is a natural manifestation of the vast Chi or fundamental energy of the universe. Just as modern science has demonstrated the elegant unity and constant inter-relationship of all matter and energy in the elemental structures and processes of our planet and the known cosmos, so too has the cumulative Chinese understanding of Chi been based on minute observation of a correspondingly delicate and interdependent web of energy patterns flowing through and forming the basis of all that exists.

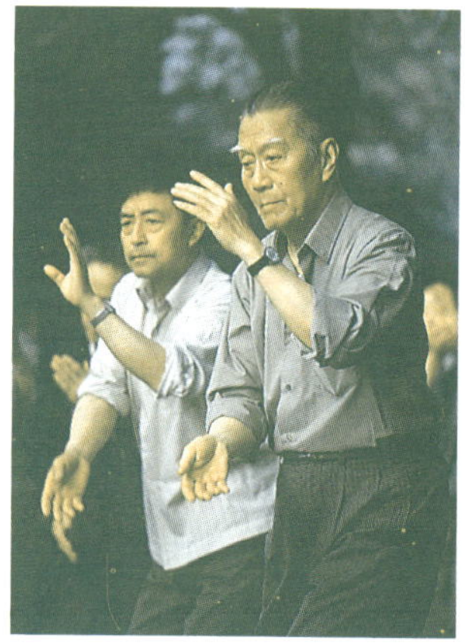

Chinese people practise Tai Chi together in local parks.

THE HUMAN ENERGY SYSTEM

One of the great contributions of early Chinese culture was the discovery that it was possible to trace and analyse very precisely the patterns of energy within the human body. This knowledge could then be used as the basis of both preventive health care and the treatment of disease.

China's most famous physicians and philosophers have contributed extensively to the analysis and practical application of the body's energy systems. From this study have come the distinctive characteristics of traditional Chinese medicine, including the practices of acupuncture and herbal medicine, and a set of exercise systems that strengthen the body internally.

Throughout the body your energy circulates along channels which in the West are called "meridians". These often run in parallel with your cardiovascular system. Through an ever finer network of radiating routes, the Chi animates the entire living matter of your body.

ENERGY BLOCKAGES

The Chi network is like any transportation system. If there is a blockage at any major point, this will automatically overload the system. In the short term, the network can usually cope with an overload by compensating in some way, but in the long term, permanent deformation or damage can occur if it persists.

Blockages in the Chi network can be caused by a range of factors. Sometimes serious disruption can be caused by bruising, muscle injuries, and sprains, especially if these are not treated properly and immediately. Long periods of sitting (common in office work and in other types of institutional work) as well as internal pressures generated by nervous tension can also block the Chi circulation. Even an extremely sedentary existence, without injury or tension, can lead to degeneration of the Chi network through irregular use or poor maintenance. Properly cared for, however, its life-enhancing properties will continue to sustain a vigorous and healthy existence for years and years.

The ancient Chinese discovered that it was possible to develop and direct the body's vital energy in particular ways. It could be nurtured to help prevent disease and premature ageing. It could be made to flow from one person to another and thereby used to help heal the sick. It could also be employed with powerful effect in the martial arts. The exercise systems used to stimulate and channel human energy came to be known as Chi Kung, which literally means "energy exercise", of which the Zhan Zhuang system is one part (see Chi Kung – the Energy Exercise, on p. 20). Some forms of Chi Kung focus exclusively on the mind, posture, breathing, or movement, or combine only some of these elements. Zhan Zhuang, the system described in this book, ultimately fuses all four together.

CHI KUNG – THE ENERGY EXERCISE

The goal of Chi Kung exercise is to stimulate the flow of energy internally in the body so that it effectively rushes through and clears the entire network of Chi channels, or "meridians".

Extensive research has been done over the years to develop a system of exercise that would speed up the blood circulation (and hence also stimulate the flow of Chi) without placing an intolerable strain on the lungs. The results drew on the accumulated wisdom of Chinese Taoist and Buddhist breathing practices and the practices and disciplines of the martial arts. Chi Kung, as the resulting exercises were known, used a series of breathing exercises to control the internal movement of Chi while the body remained virtually motionless.

For centuries most knowledge about Chi Kung was passed on within families or small circles of masters and students and kept relatively secret. It is only recently that it has been taught and discussed publicly. There are a growing number of applications of Chi Kung exercise, ranging from the treatment of chronic illness through to the development of extraordinary physical powers that enable practitioners to break stones with their bare fingers. Now, it is increasingly being used to assist in the treatment of illnesses that Western medical practice cannot treat successfully. It is also being used to help prevent illness by building up the body's immune systems and internal strength. What Chi Kung offers is a method of training the nervous system, the mind, and the internal organs simultaneously, so that the inner strength of the whole person is raised to a new level of power and fitness.

ONE DESTINATION, MANY ROUTES

There are many styles and schools of Chi Kung. There is Chi Kung for health, for therapy, for martial arts, and for spiritual development. There are Buddhist and Taoist schools of Chi Kung. In the martial arts, Chi Kung training includes techniques known as "iron palm", "iron shirt", and "metal bell cover". In athletics Chi Kung is used to develop muscle power and endurance. In medicine, especially in China, there are two main branches of Chi Kung: one is moving Chi Kung which involves movement exercise; the other is limited to static breathing and meditational exercises.

In the spiritual field, there are Chi Kung exercises that enable the student to experience other dimensions, and to develop telepathic powers.

The goal, however, of building internal strength, remains fundamental to all.

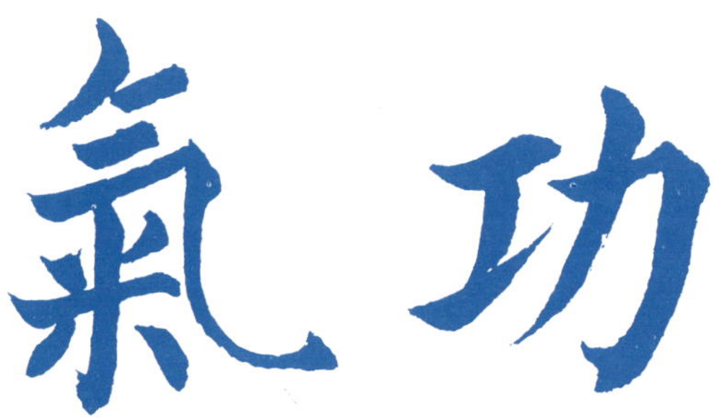

Chi Kung

The ability to transform energy and even create it within you is one of the profound secrets of life. Like a tree, you are one of the great power-stations of nature. You share a deep affinity with the countless trees and saplings that surround you on the planet. They have much to teach us. They are perfectly adapted to the rhythm of the seasons. They combine immense strength with the most delicate sensitivity. They turn sunlight and air into fuel. They share the earth with others, but are secure within themselves.

This is the vision of life so beautifully expressed in the ancient Taoist classic of Lao Tzu, the Tao Teh Ching:

> Standing alone and unchanging,
>
> One can observe every mystery,
>
> Present at every moment and ceaselessly continuing –
>
> This is the gateway to indescribable marvels.

This is one of the earliest references to Zhan Zhuang. You are standing like a tree, alone and unmoving. You come to understand everything that happens within you – all the internal changes that take place in your organs and muscles. You practise constantly. You feel the reactions taking place. The feeling never stops. It goes on and on, over and over again. This is the Way: no matter how far you go you will never come to the end of all the wondrous things there are to discover.

站樁

Zhan Zhuang

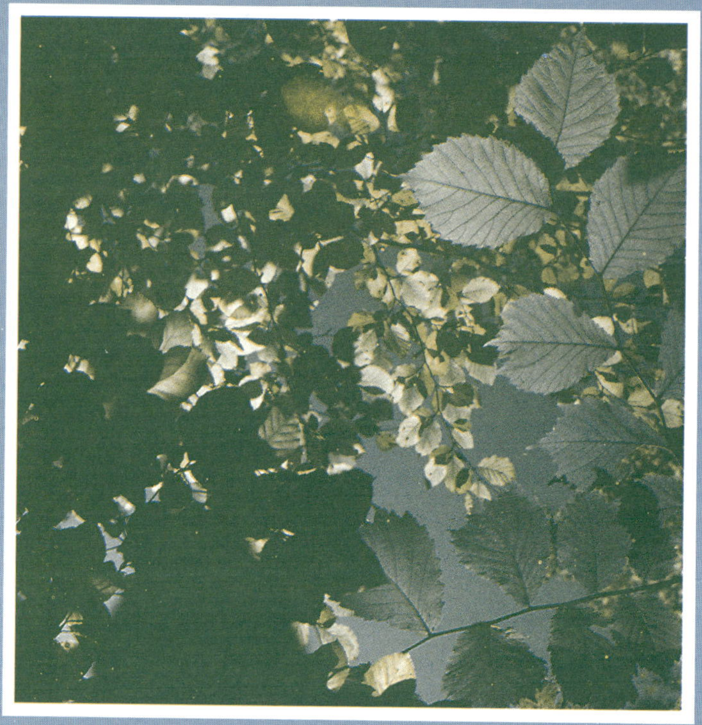

PART ONE

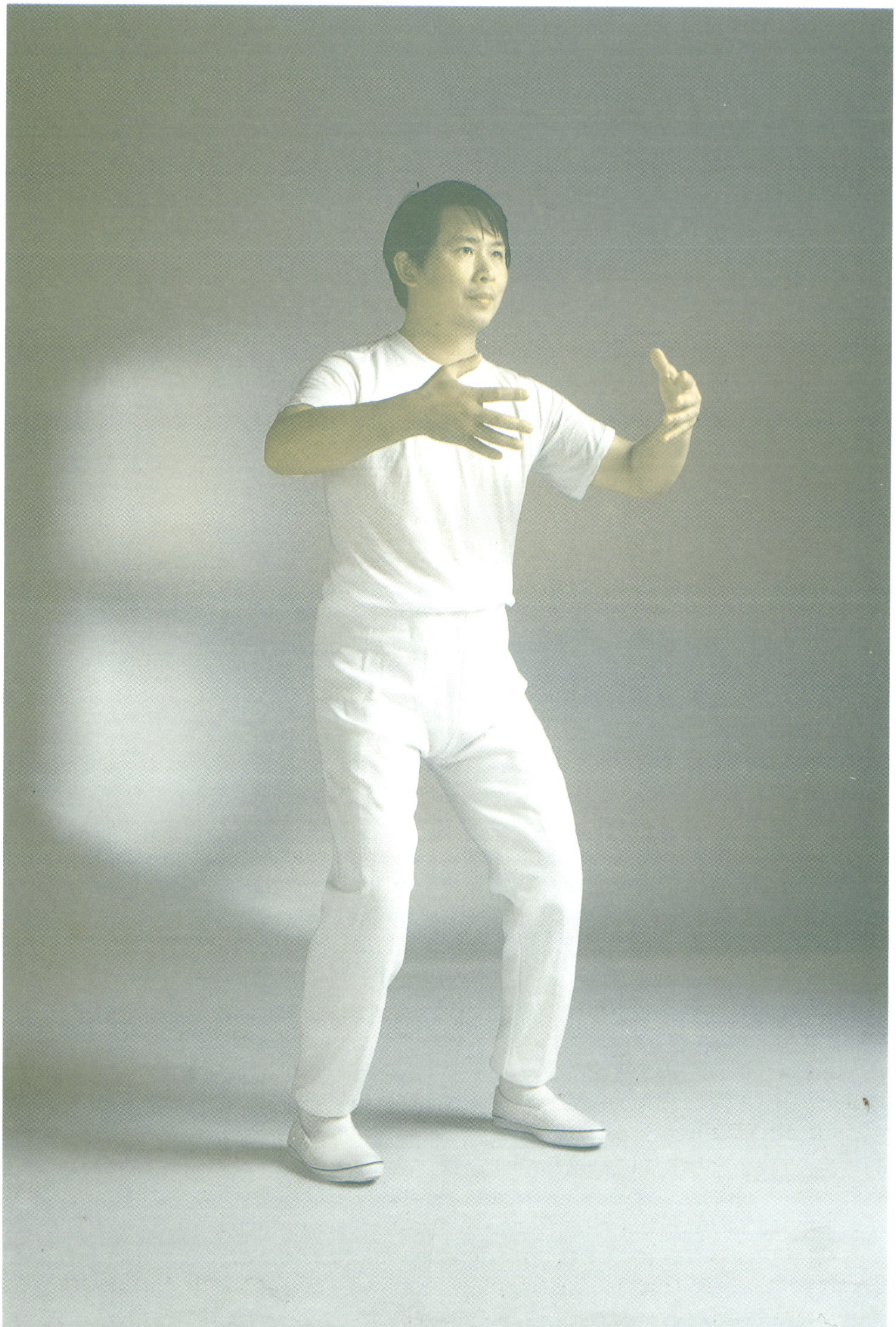

Master Lam in the second position.

CHAPTER 1
LEARNING TO STAND

The Zhan Zhuang system begins with two basic standing exercises. These start to build up and release the natural flow of energy inside you. The first position, a simple standing posture (pp. 28-29), enables you to relax your body in preparation for the other exercises. The second position, "Holding the Balloon" (pp. 34-35), is the key position in the whole system. It is essential to become thoroughly comfortable in both these positions before moving on to the exercises in Part Two, the intermediate level.

The simple warm up routines on the following pages prepare your body for the internal changes that take place during the Zhan Zhuang exercises. They are essential for beginners, because although the standing positions do not look strenuous, if you do them properly the resulting activity inside your body is enormous, and affects your whole system.

During the exercises in this chapter you may feel a little weak, start to tremble, or begin to tense up. But don't move: breathe naturally and relax. Use the time to notice all the remarkable changes and sensations in your body. Remember: standing still is not doing nothing, it *is* the exercise.

When you are familiar with the first two standing exercises, you will need to learn how to breathe and relax, as described in Chapter 2. This will give you the experience of simultaneous exertion and relaxation during the standing postures, which is fundamental to this exercise system. The curious sensations you are likely to experience when you begin the exercises are described in Chapter 3.

Start by doing the standing exercises for five minutes a day. After three weeks, increase this to ten minutes. Three weeks later, aim for 15 minutes, and 20 minutes after a further three weeks. You can stand for longer if you wish, but 20 minutes will refresh your whole system. Follow the step-by-step advice, practising a little every day. Do not skip ahead: developing self-control is part of the training.

Warming up

As with all exercise routines, the warm up is essential. It helps your body become flexible and helps open up the internal channels along which your energy flows. The two largest and most important joints are the knees and shoulders. So by loosening these up first you are most likely to get the rich benefits of the later Zhan Zhuang exercises.

As a beginner, it is important to do these warm up exercises every time you start your Zhan Zhuang practice. They will take you about six or seven minutes.

Regularly practised, they give long-term protection against arthritis and other painful ailments that reduce the original flexibility of the body. If you are an advanced student (for example, if you have practised Tai Chi Chuan for several years), you can warm up instead with the Ba Duan Jin system described in Chapter 4.

WHEN AND WHERE TO PRACTISE

First thing in the morning before eating is the best time to begin. At other times, allow half an hour after meals before starting the exercise.

Try to do the exercises where the air is fresh – outside is ideal, but a well-ventilated, quiet room is next best.

CLOTHING

Make sure you are relaxed and comfortable. Wear loose clothing while training. Otherwise, loosen your collar and belt, and remove your wristwatch. Don't train in tight trousers or jeans, or wearing high-heeled shoes.

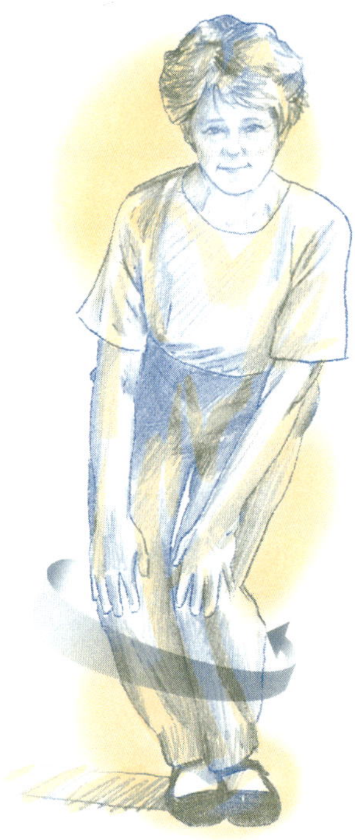

WARMING UP YOUR KNEES

The first warm up is for your knees. During the exercise, try to remain relaxed from your waist up. To avoid tension in your neck, look slightly down to a point about 2m (6ft) in front of you. For added benefit from this exercise, double the number of circles.

Stand with your feet together. Bend your knees and stoop over so that you can just touch them with your fingers. With your hands on your knees, rotate your knees 30 times to the left (see left) and 30 times to the right.

LOOSENING YOUR SHOULDERS

The second warm up is for your shoulders. Make 30 to 40 complete circles with your arms. You should start very slowly, then speed up slightly, and then slow down again toward the end. Do 60 circles for greater benefit.

Breathe in as your arms come up. Breathe out as they come down. If you are short of breath, breathe in and out as your arms come up, and in and out as they come down.

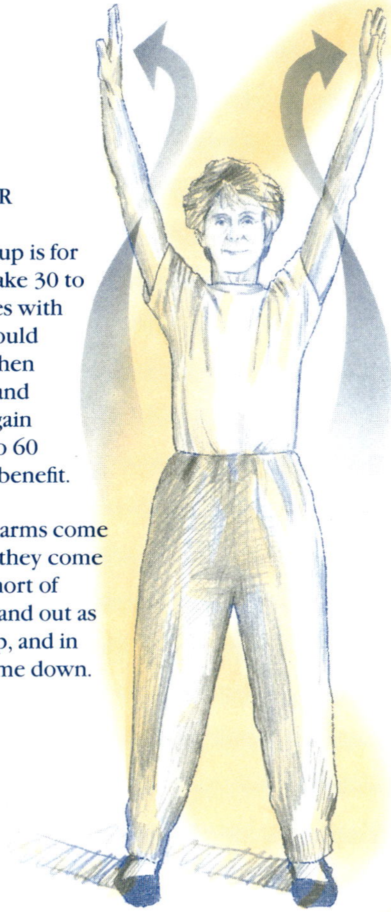

1. Stand with your feet a shoulder-width apart, toes pointing forward. Slowly raise your arms as if you were holding a large beach ball between your palms. When your hands are above the top of your head, turn them outward.

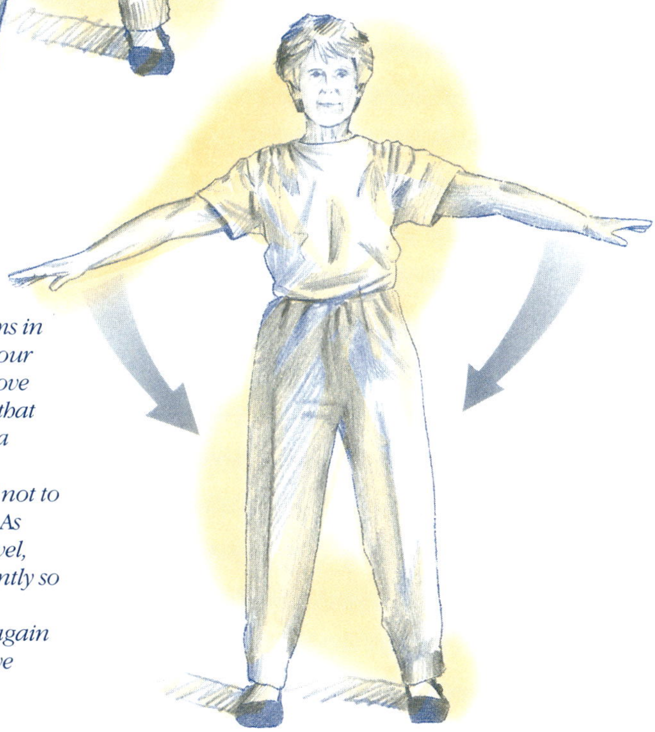

2. Then lower your arms in an arc down toward your sides. As your hands move slowly down, imagine that each is gently pressing a smaller beach ball downward. Be careful not to hunch your shoulders. As your arms reach hip level, bring them forward gently so that they can hold the imaginary beach ball again before they start to move slowly upward.

Wu Chi – the first position

All Zhan Zhuang training begins with this position, which is profoundly important. Even at extraordinarily advanced levels of exercise, we begin with a period of quiet standing in the Wu Chi position – the position of primal energy.

The Wu Chi position involves simply standing still. It is an opportunity to pay careful attention to the tensions in your body and its nervous system. At the same time it becomes a moment of powerful, deep relaxation in your day. Simple as it may seem, this opening position, correctly practised, holds the key to unlock the storehouse of your great internal energy reserves.

It is a good idea to go to the toilet before starting, to ensure that you do not have to interrupt your stationary exercise.

Try to do your training outside, with your back toward the sun. If you can stand near a large tree with the sun on your back, this is the best location of all. Don't stand in the rain or fog.

If you're indoors, you can either use a quiet room or create a tranquil environment by playing a recording of softly flowing instrumental music.

MOVING INTO THE POSITION

Stand with your feet a shoulder-width apart, toes pointing forward, either parallel, or turned slightly outward. Let your hands hang loosely by your sides and drop your shoulders. Imagine that, like a puppet, your whole body is hanging, suspended from your head. A string holds your head from a point at the top of your skull, directly in line with the tips of your ears. Feel yourself sinking down, relaxing, as you hang from the string.

Breathe calmly and naturally. Stand quietly, allowing your whole system to calm down, for up to five minutes. As you do this, mentally follow through the points on the illustration (right), starting at the top of your head. Study it carefully and make sure that you pay meticulous attention to all the elements presented in it. Return to these points again and again until you are able to assume the Wu Chi position naturally and perfectly.

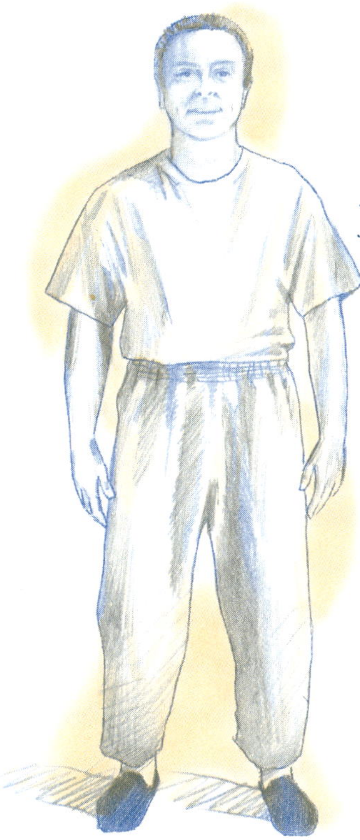

Your eyes look forward and slightly downward.

Drop your chin a little so that your throat is not pushed forward. Release any tension in your neck.

Let your arms hang loosely. Drop your shoulders and your elbows.

Relax your hips and belly. Let the bottom of your spine unfold downward so that neither your belly nor your bottom is sticking out.

Stand with your heels at least a shoulder-width apart. Never stand pigeon-toed.

Inhale and exhale gently through your nose only. Your mouth should be closed, but not tightly shut. Don't clamp your teeth shut. If saliva forms, swallow it.

Exhale completely and allow your chest to drop: this is the ideal posture.

Don't stiffen your fingers. Allow them to curve gently and remain slightly apart.

Unlock your knees. You can bend them ever so slightly. Make sure they don't stiffen into the fixed, locked position.

THE FIRST POSITION

PRACTICE TIME

At first, even this simplest of all things – just standing still for a few minutes – may seem impossible when you try it. Thirty seconds may seem like an eternity; five minutes may be agony. The boredom may drive you crazy. These reactions are simply the evidence of the constant tension in your nervous system and proof that you need this exercise. Zhan Zhuang has started to alert you to the confused patterns of energy in your body.

Aligning mind and body

When you stand still in the first position, with your body correctly aligned, you are drawing energy (Chi) from the earth, and accelerating its flow through your body. This practice of standing still is an ancient discipline. The first known reference to it dates back to the oldest and most influential book in the history of world medicine, *The Yellow Emperor's Classic of Internal Medicine* (Huang Ti Nei Ching), thought to have been written about 4,000 years ago. In the opening section, the Emperor tells the court physician:

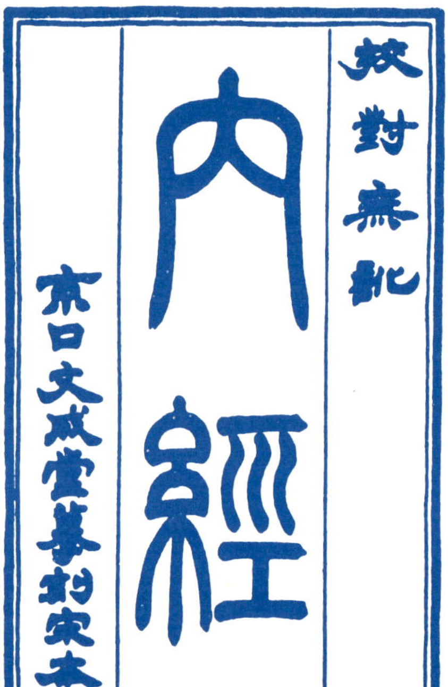

I have heard that in ancient times there were the so-called Spiritual Beings:

They stood between Heaven and Earth, connecting the Universe;

They understood and were able to control both Yin and Yang, the two fundamental principles of nature;

They inhaled the vital essence of life;

They remained unmoving in their spirit;

Their muscles and flesh were as one –

This is the Tao, the Way you are looking for.

Illustration from the title page of The Yellow Emperor's Classic of Internal Medicine.

This poetic passage refers to "standing still without changing", which we now call Zhan Zhuang. You stand aligned between the ground and the sky, connecting the two great forces of heaven and earth. You are able to understand the fundamental forces of energy in your body. When you practise in this way, with the full force of your spirit, not only will your whole body and mind be synchronized, but you will have the feeling that heaven and earth are fused together through you.

YING AND YANG
Yin and Yang are opposite and complementary forces such as day and night, female and male, in our ever-changing universe. The theory of Yin and Yang, fundamental to Chinese medicine, is described in the Yellow Emperor's classic work.

Adjusting your position

When you become comfortable in this position, think about the points below. Quietly adjust your body to correct your balance and position.

The point from which you are suspended is in line with the tips of your ears.

Your whole frame is suspended from the top of your head. You hang from it like a puppet, or a garment on a coat hanger.

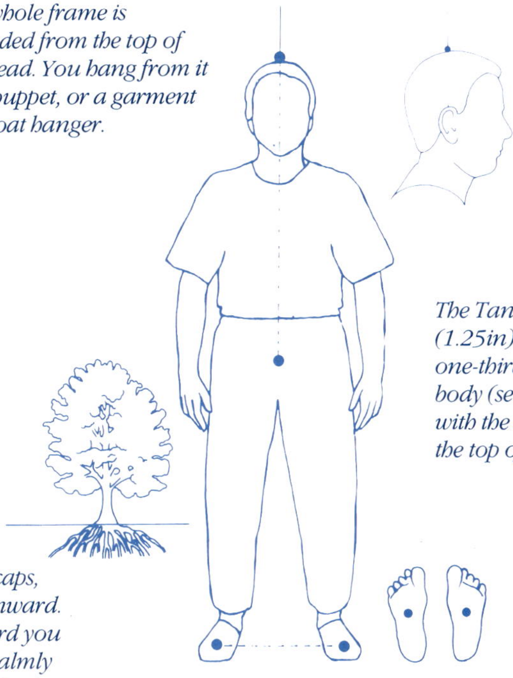

The Tan Tien lies 3cm (1.25in) below your navel, one-third of the way into your body (see p. 42). It is in line with the suspension point at the top of your head.

From below your kneecaps, your roots extend downward. From your knees upward you rise like a tree, resting calmly between the earth and the sky.

Your weight is evenly distributed between your left and right feet. These roots sink deep into the earth, like those of a tree.

The weight of your body rests in the middle of the soles of your feet.

A FIELD OF ENERGY

The Chinese like to exercise in the presence of trees, whose Chi is wonderful. Trees are totally exposed to the elements and draw their power from everything around them. They reach deep into the soil with their roots. They reach upward toward the light. Their fibrous trunks are filled with the flow of life. They take strength from the earth, from water and rain, from the sun, from the air, and from the space that surrounds them. This is what we have in mind when we say "stand like a tree". You are a field of energy. You are nourished by everything around you, like a tree standing in the midst of all the elements.

The Tree in Winter

This is the time of hidden regeneration. Mist hangs above the ground. Frost forms on open fields.

The tree is still. It stands alone and quiet. In the darkness of the early morning, nature is asleep. There is no movement in the air, no hint of trembling in the branches. The tree is silent in the darkness like a stone – a pillar in the courtyard of an empty temple.

A distant sound breaks through the stillness. The day's first light advances on the earth. The shadow of the tree moves with the dawn, but the tree is motionless.

The ground beneath the tree is frozen hard. Above the ground, the bark is cold, the limbs are stiff. A passer-by might wonder if the tree will live in spring.

But underneath the ground the earth is warm. The weight of all the tree sinks to its roots. They are indifferent to the frozen soil, they grow toward the centre of the earth.

The tree is not afraid. It was a seed: it knows the earth is holding it. Within its core, a vital ring is being formed. Around its spine, new life is rising from the earth, while flakes of snow are settling on the silent and unmoving tree.

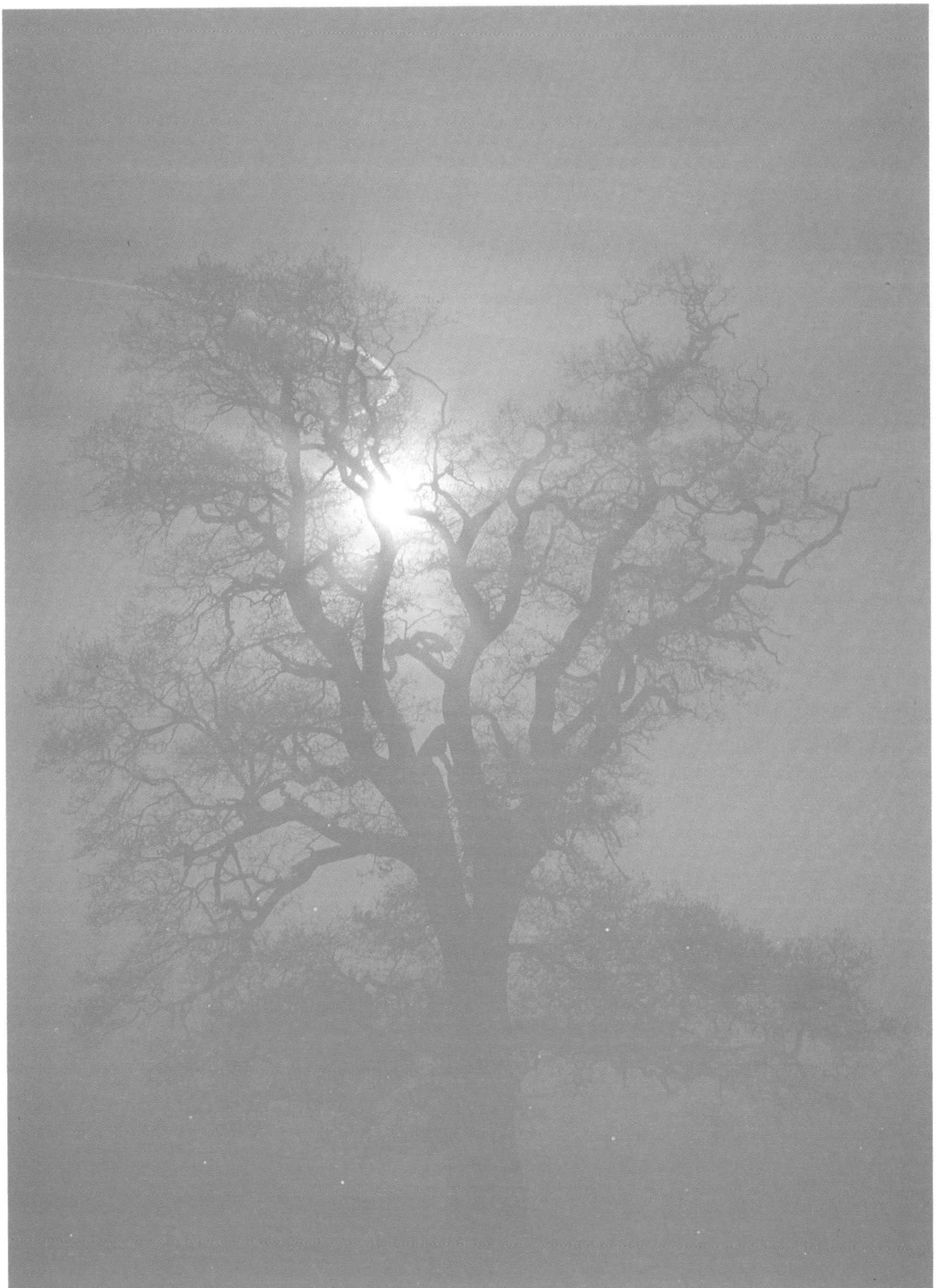

Holding the balloon – the second position

The next step in Zhan Zhuang training is to start "Holding the Balloon". This position forms the basis for many of the more advanced exercises, and speeds the inner circulation of energy through your feet, up through your entire body, and to your hands and head.

Try holding the second position for up to five minutes. You will probably experience considerable pain from the tension in your shoulders, arms, and knees. This is partly muscle fatigue, partly the reaction of your nervous system. Be patient. Nothing you are doing is harmful. You are returning to an original state of being. Your journey will take discipline and diligence.

As you hold this position, imagine that you are resting on a series of other balloons that take your full weight (see right).

To begin with, as you stand quietly holding the imaginary balloon, review all the guidelines for this position (see right).

MOVING INTO THE POSITION

From the first position, the Wu Chi position (see p. 29), sink down slightly. Your knees bend as you sink downward. Your head, torso, and pelvic girdle remain gently aligned, exactly as they were in the first position. Your spine unfolds downward and straightens naturally. Do not bend forward. Imagine you are simply resting your bottom on the edge of a high stool. Your weight rests equally on both feet.

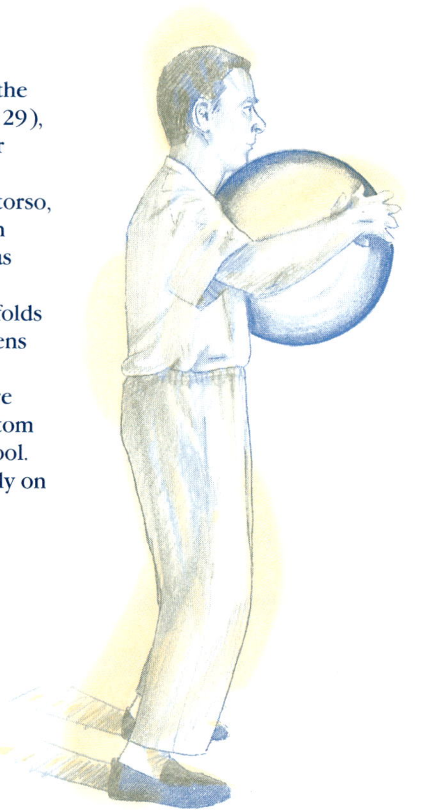

1. Slowly bring both your arms upward and forward to form an open circle in front of your chest at about shoulder level. Your open palms face your chest.

The distance between the fingertips of your hands is the equivalent of one to three fists, 7-21cm (3-9in). The tops of your thumbs are no higher than your shoulders. Your wrists are as wide apart as your shoulders. Your elbows are slightly lower than your wrists and shoulders. The inner angle between your upper arm and forearm is slightly more than 90 degrees.

2. Imagine that you are holding a large inflated balloon between your hands, forearms, and chest. You are gently keeping it in place without tension. It is resting naturally on the inner surface of the circle formed by your fingers, palms, arms, and chest.

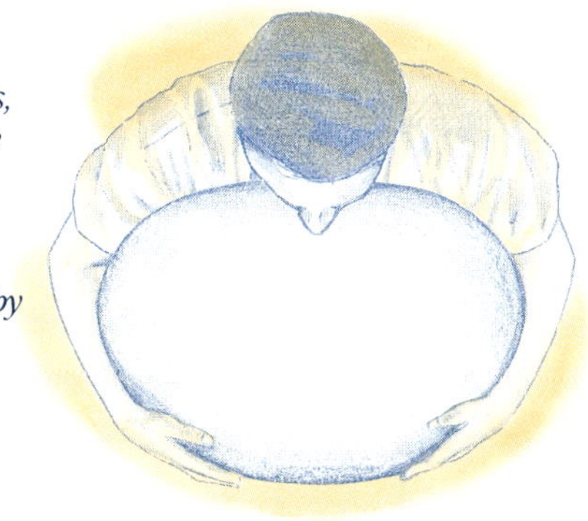

Your armpits and upper arms rest on two small balloons.

Your elbows rest on two large balloons that float on the surface of a pond.

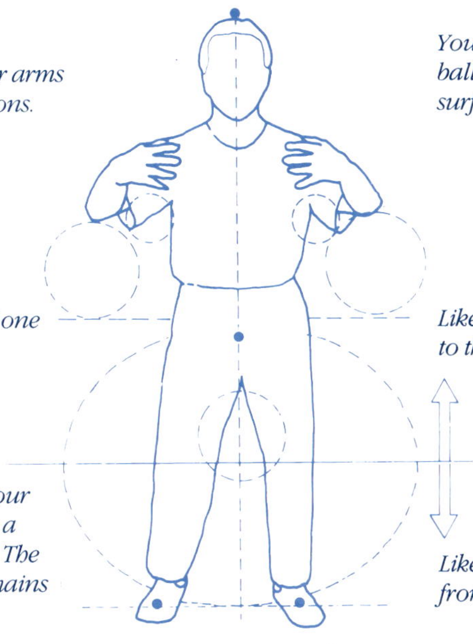

Your thighs gently hold one balloon in place.

Like a tree you reach upward to the sky.

A huge balloon takes your weight behind you, like a beach ball on the sand. The weight on your feet remains slightly forward.

Like a tree you are rooted from below.

RESTING ON IMAGINARY BALLOONS

VISUALIZING THE BALLOONS

The balloons are an indispensable element of this remarkable system. You must visualize them clearly in your mind. By holding the imaginary balloon in your arms you release any pressure constricting the sides of your chest and abdomen. Maintaining the position builds up both your physical and mental stamina. You begin to place carefully balanced, but increasing, demands on your energy and blood systems that step up the circulation in both. The other imaginary balloons are a powerful aid to relaxation; learn to sink fully into them.

The Tree in Blossom

The season changes imperceptibly. The early morning light is pale. Clouds drift on the horizon. In the distance nothing moves. The dawn is still.

The tree remains unmoving, but is changed.

The morning air is warm, the grass is moist. The tiny creatures of the soil are moving in the ground.

The tree's roots stretch their new growth in the earth – alive to countless changes in their dark and humid world. Their slender filaments draw in the silent dew that glistens in the soil.

The earth is rising through the tree. Inside its mighty trunk, life trembles and awakens.

Immense, alone, the tree is giving birth. New shoots are opening in the air. Curled leaves emerge in miniature – the work of winter's still and solitary months.

The tree is utterly consumed in growth. Its bark is stretched. Innumerable cells are giving birth.

The morning winds sweep through the spreading tree. On every branch the buds and blossoms tremble in the breeze. The growing leaves reach out to every sunbeam. The leaves' open pores are breathing and their veins are full.

The tree is wreathed in silence like a waterfall. It stands transfixed: poised motionless between the mighty pull of all its tiny root hairs and the fragrant, evanescent petals on its boughs.

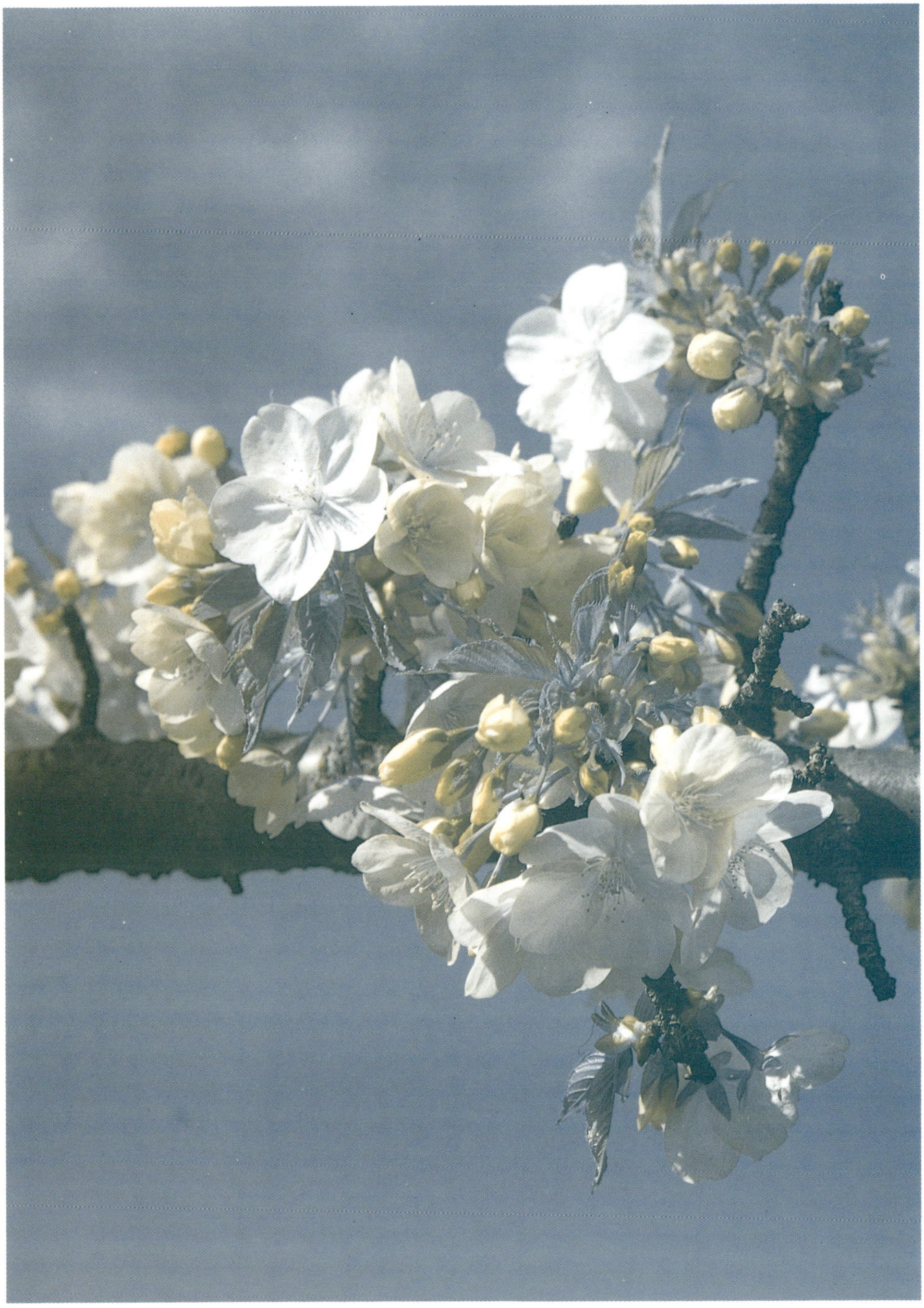

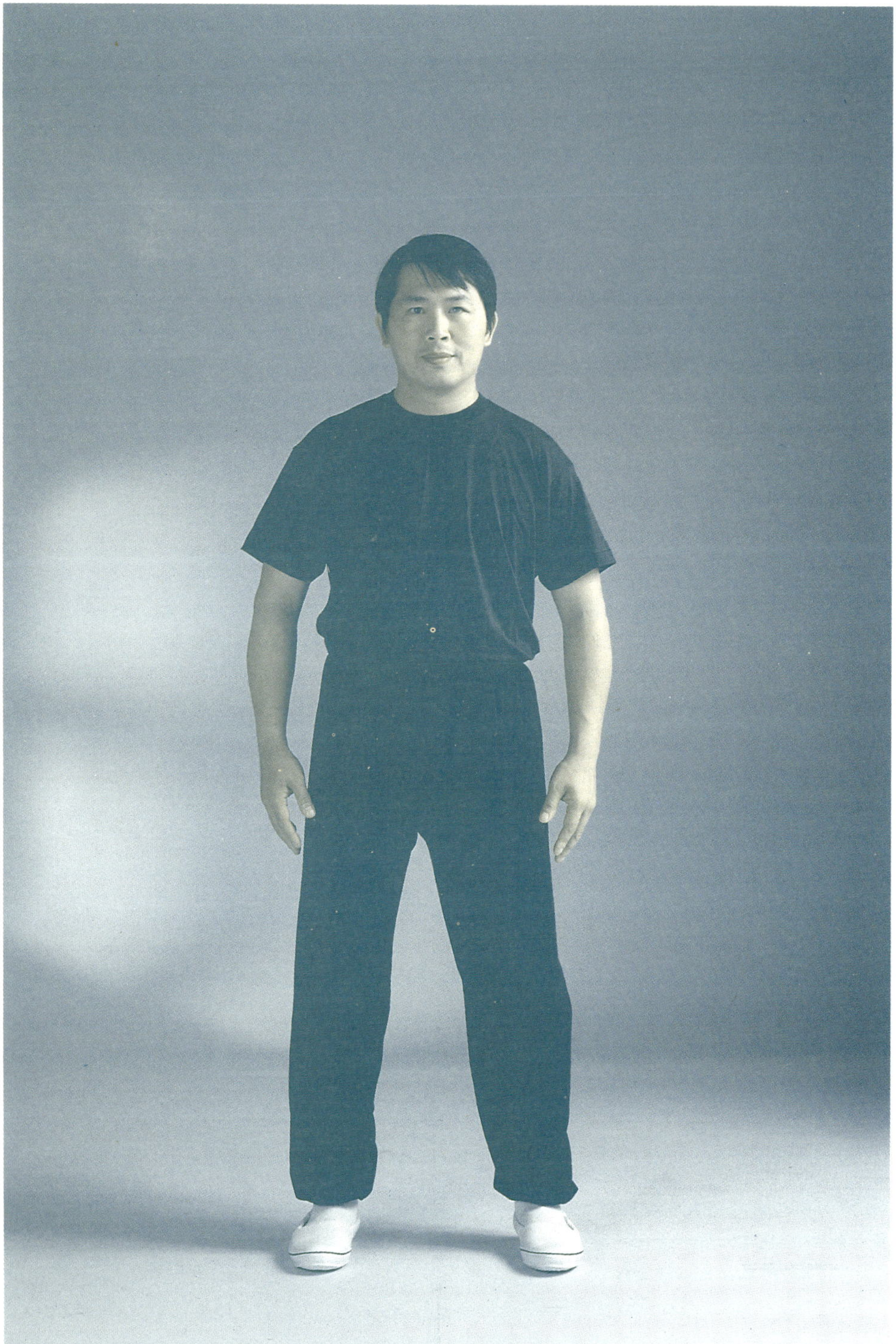

Master Lam in the first position.

Practical tips

The benefits of Zhan Zhuang practice result from inner growth and transformation. The fundamental changes begin to occur in your internal organs and nervous system. Without unusual sensitivity or training, most of us cannot sense these at first, whereas we can all feel the immediate effect of hard muscular activity such as jogging or weight training. The initial impact of Zhan Zhuang takes place deep inside you, like an explosion in the depths of the sea, and so it is all the more important to be aware of what to do when you start your training.

Points To Remember

- *If you feel tired or faint, don't close your eyes, otherwise you might risk falling down.*
- *Remind yourself to relax while holding the correct position. You will need to check for tension over and over again.*
- *When you finish the second position, lower your arms and stand quietly for two or three minutes. Then gently shake your arms and legs. Then it's a good idea to make a final series of 20 circles with your arms at moderate speed.*
- *Finally, walk around slowly for a couple of minutes. You are then ready for the day!*
- *Women: your increased blood circulation may make your periods heavier. In this case, stand for less than 20 minutes during menstruation.*

YOUR APPEARANCE

After you have finished your standing exercise it is a good idea to rub your hands several times over your face, as if you were giving yourself a wash. This increases the flow of Chi in your hands and the circulation of Chi through your facial skin. You will look fresher – almost "polished"! This, combined with increased alertness, will give your eyes a clearer and brighter look.

CHECKING YOURSELF

Two simple tests show that the exercises are making changes in your body.

Stand with your feet a shoulder-width apart. Leave one arm loosely by your side. Raise your other arm into the second Zhan Zhuang position, as if you were holding a large balloon between that arm and your chest. Breathe slowly from the Tan Tien several times (see p. 42). After one or two minutes you will feel the difference in your right and left sides. Then, raise your other arm to hold another balloon. You can feel the energy circuit without your fingers touching!

To feel the increased circulation, try a second test. Stand for 10-15 minutes, holding the invisible balloon between your hands and chest. Then, lower your arms. The tingling sensation in your fingers is the result of the rush of blood and Chi.

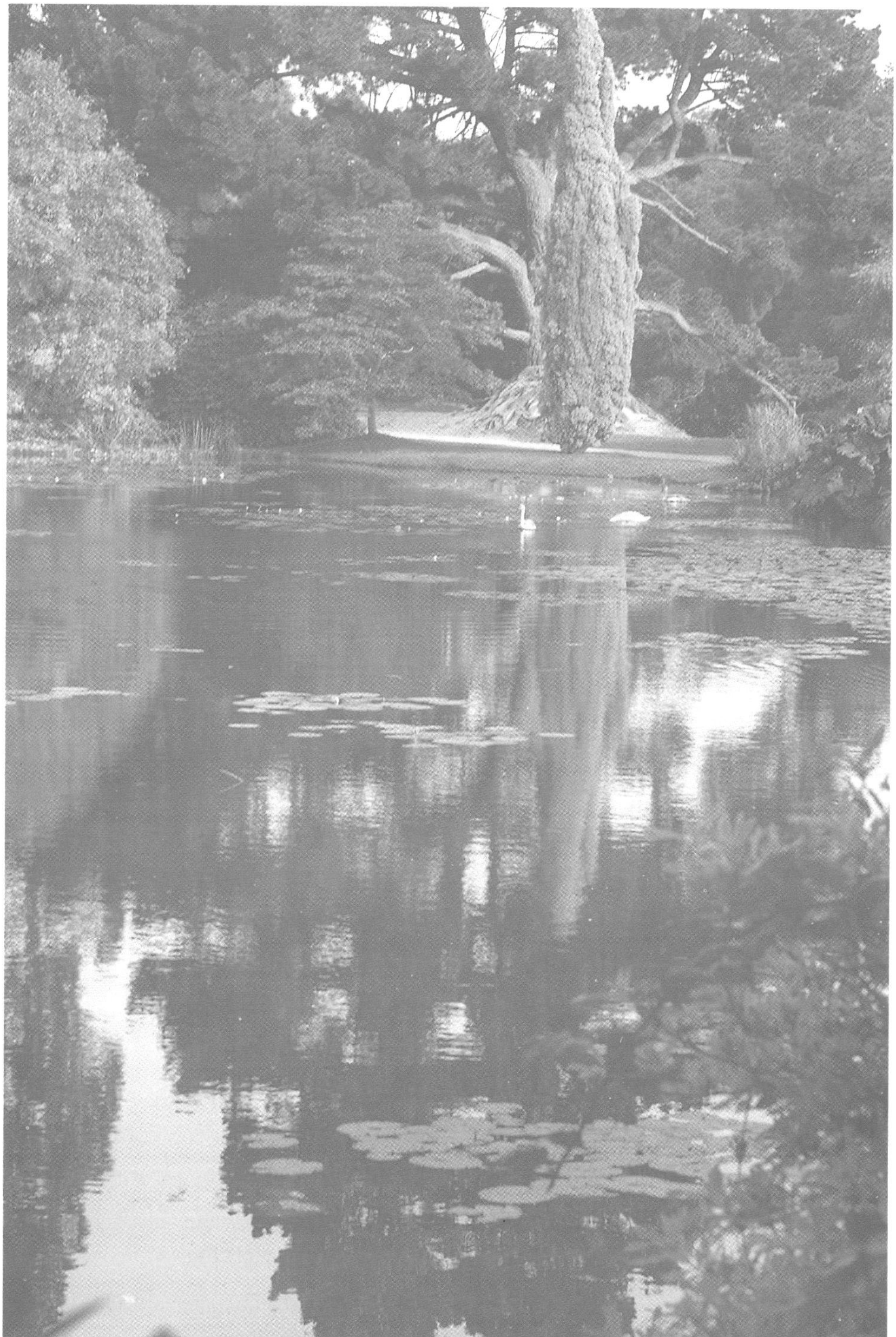

CHAPTER 2
BREATHING AND RELAXING

Think of a baby in the womb. The gently curved positions of Zhan Zhuang are based on that original state. They enable your energy to redirect itself properly through the curves of your major joints. But there are two other elements that are vital to the rediscovery of your original, natural energy. These are your breath, and the condition of your mental and nervous systems.

The state of your mental and nervous systems has a profound effect on your breathing and the functioning of your entire being. Thoughts and feelings have obvious effects on your respiration and your heartbeat. They have a powerful influence on the chemicals released into your bloodstream and on the tension in your muscles. A classic example of this is the effect of worry on the heartbeat, the breathing rate, and the digestive system. These same effects can be detrimental to your Chi system, blocking the flow of energy through your body, and restricting your ability to absorb and utilize the universal Chi that surrounds you every moment of your life.

Over the centuries various techniques have been developed to help people calm their minds. Some methods advise you to concentrate your mind on one point or to follow the rise and fall of your breathing without allowing yourself to be distracted. Other meditational systems are based on repeating a word or phrase so that your mind comes to focus solely on that activity and slowly lets go of other preoccupations.

Because of the tremendous mental effort they require, these systems often increase the level of tension in both the body and the mind. Many of them focus exclusively on the mental aspect and neglect the rest of the human organism. In Zhan Zhuang training, the aim is to train your mind and body at the same time. The training includes what the Chinese call "mentality exercises" – using the efforts of your mind to relax the muscles in your body. Like other systems, this takes a lot of care initially; but in the end, your Chi will flow through a relaxed body that is synchronized with a relaxed mind.

Breathing

Most young people and adults breathe by raising and opening the chest cavity. Many people who do conventional fitness exercises and take part in strenuous sports breathe from the chest as well. This is how their breathing has developed in the years since birth. Our goal is different, however. We want to return to the powerful, deep breathing we were born with, in order to enhance the power of our vitality.

Natural breathing is centred on the Tan Tien inside your abdomen (see below). This way of breathing is very different from the shallow, quick action that is common in people who breathe only with the chest. Breathing from the Tan Tien refocuses your energy in the original centre of your body through which you were nourished before birth.

Unlike many other systems, Zhan Zhuang does not insist on special breathing: the emphasis in Zhan Zhuang training is placed on the power of the mind to control the body. If you find that trying the abdominal breathing described below distracts you from standing calmly, return to your normal breathing.

TAN TIEN BREATHING

To begin with, you should practise the following exercise for several minutes before standing in the Zhan Zhuang positions.

Stand with your feet a shoulder-width apart, toes pointing forward. Fold your hands over your abdomen, putting your right thumb over your navel and resting your left hand on top of your right hand. Keep your mouth gently closed: do not clench your teeth.

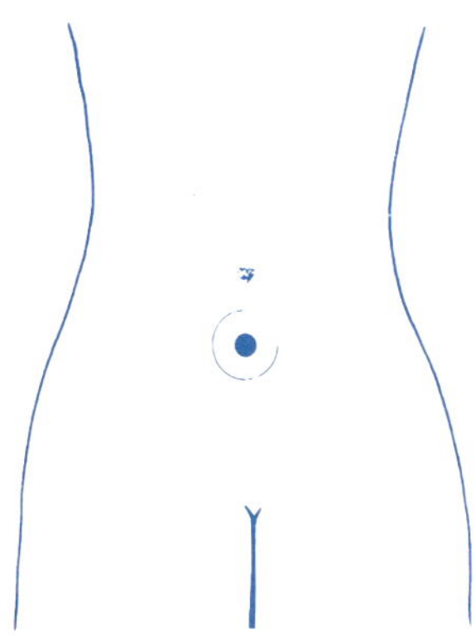

The Tan Tien lies 3cm (1.25in) below your navel, one-third of the way into your body. It is in line with the suspension point at the top of your head, when you are standing in any one of the Zhan Zhuang positions.

HINTS FOR BEGINNERS

As a beginner, you can use your hands to help establish the correct belly movement. Press in slightly as you breathe out. As you breathe in, feel your belly filling up under your hand. You can practise Tan Tien breathing with your eyes open or closed, but avoid staring with your eyes fixed open as this will generate tension. If you have trouble relaxing, place a glass of water on a table a few feet in front of you and look at it while you stand.

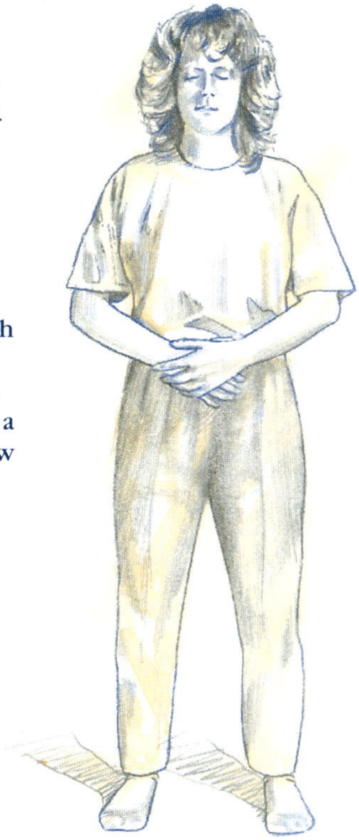

Quietly and slowly breathe out through your nose. As you exhale, draw your belly in so that you feel you are squeezing the air out of your torso from the bottom up. Breathe out smoothly and soundlessly, until you feel you have emptied your lungs.

When you are ready to breathe in, inhale through your nose and allow your belly to expand outward as if the incoming air is filling your abdomen. Allow this to happen naturally: don't force your belly out. Just let the air filter in smoothly and steadily without tension.

REFINING THE TECHNIQUE

Once Tan Tien breathing becomes a habit, and you incorporate it into your Zhan Zhuang training, only concentrate on breathing out. If you concentrate on breathing in, you will tend to tense up. If you concentrate on your outgoing breath it will help you relax and your inward breath will automatically have a natural, full flow.

Calming your mind and body

The Zhan Zhuang system works on the mind in two ways: some of the exercises calm the mind; others aim to strengthen the power of the mind. You cannot accomplish the second without having achieved the first. Therefore, anyone starting Zhan Zhuang training must first work on calming the mind. Ultimately, you need to develop your mental control to the point where your mind can make your body relax precisely at the moment that your whole system is subjected to the greatest possible stress on it. This makes Zhan Zhuang one of the most personally demanding exercise systems ever developed. It requires an extraordinarily high level of synchronization between the mind and body. To begin this, direct your mind through your body, by following the instructions below.

SMILE TO RELAX

To begin the mental exercise, start at the top of your body. Once you have adopted one of the first two Zhan Zhuang positions, think of your face. Think of smiling and then feel your facial muscles relax as a gentle smile begins to form. Feel your eyes, cheek muscles, and lips lose their tension as you begin to smile.

CHECK YOUR BREATH

Then make sure you are breathing from the Tan Tien (see p. 42). Make sure you are paying attention to your outgoing breath only, and then allowing yourself to inhale effortlessly. Once this becomes automatic, you should ignore your breathing altogether.

RELAX YOUR BODY

Having relaxed your face and checked your breathing, use your mind to travel through your body from top to toe, relaxing every joint and sinew. Begin at the very top of your head and work down from your skull to your neck, to your right and left shoulders, to your elbows, wrists, and fingers. Then continue down through your ribs and backbone to your pelvic girdle and then through your thighs and knees to your ankles and toes. As your mind makes its slow journey downward, search for tension and tell each muscle group to relax. You can talk silently to yourself: "Now I am reaching my left shoulder... I want it to relax... Now it is relaxed... I can move on..." and so forth, following the route of your entire skeleton.

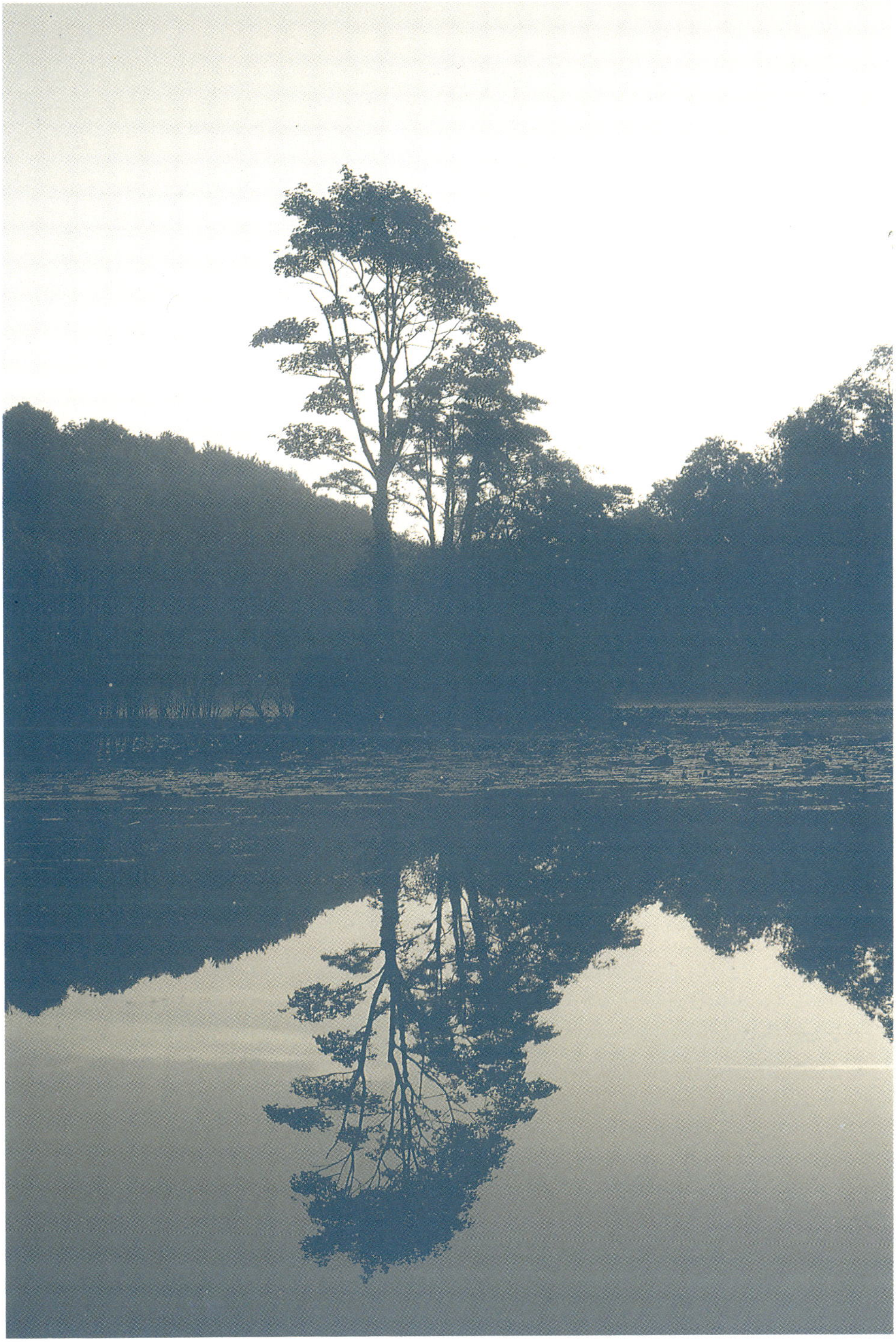

Staying relaxed

As explained earlier in this chapter, the very first step in Zhan Zhuang is to train your body to relax. By systematically relaxing your body from top to toe you start the process not only of calming your mind but also of increasing the ability of your mind to focus on relaxation. In this way, although you are working, your mind is at rest. Even this can prove difficult to sustain for long, since your mind must continue to order your straining muscles to relax, and carry you through the initial stages of pain. Just thinking about relaxing can make you tense! So, if you are having trouble in the early stages, here are some techniques that may help you. Try these while standing in the second position, Holding the Balloon (pp. 34-35).

QUIETENING YOUR MIND

1. Thoughts, images, sounds, and your internal dialogue will still be coming and going. If anything, you will be even more aware of them. That awareness in itself is an essential development. Just use it to note what is going on in your mind. Don't worry about the fact that your mind is moving: observe whatever happens (you can even make a mental note – "Now I'm thinking...") and let it pass naturally.

2. Try standing when you are very sleepy – just before going to bed or very early in the morning. Your mind will be relatively dull, and as you stand still you will find that the whole exercise takes far less effort. Carry that feeling of relaxation with you and see if you can return to it the next time you stand in an alert state.

3. If you have trouble standing for the full time you have set yourself and you find you are starting to think about giving up, start counting slowly down, say from 200 to 0. Just keep track of the numbers; everything else – the pain, the boredom, and the time – will take care of itself.

4. If you find you worry a lot about how many minutes you have been standing or have left to go, try finding a soothing piece of music that lasts the length of time you plan to stand. Put it on, listen to it, relax your muscles from time to time, and stop when the music stops. Or you can try the Chinese way, which is to light a stick of incense and stand until it goes out. The aroma will have a soothing effect and with a little experimentation you will know how long you have been standing. You can start with a short stick at the beginning and gradually work up to a longer one.

5. If you feel unbearable pain from tension in your arms (described in more detail on page 49 and in chapter 3), put all your imagination to work to visualize the balloons that support you (see p. 35). Imagine they are floating on water: its buoyancy and the air in the balloons will easily take your weight!

6. If your feet are tense, grip the floor with your toes for a little while.

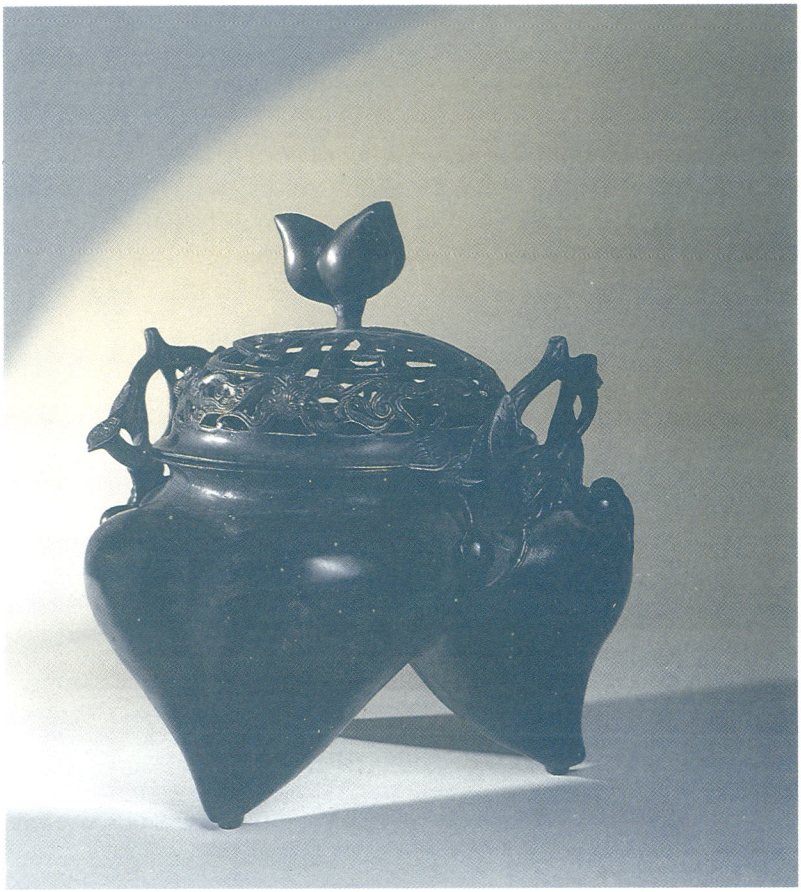

Antique Chinese incense burner, designed to reflect the shape of a peach, symbolic of eternal vitality.

7. If you feel that your bent legs can no longer support you, that is the moment to visualize the huge balloon on which you are sitting. Even if you drop all your weight into it, the air inside it can support you effortlessly.

8. As you feel the tension easing in your legs and feet, try imagining that you are standing on a soft cotton cloth that gently absorbs all your body weight.

9. If you find tension persists, there are suggestions on the next pages to help you rest while standing. Gradually, you will come to feel that you are being mysteriously supported in place. Just as you swayed peacefully in the womb before birth, now you will be lazily resting in the air. You will be ready for the next stage of the training.

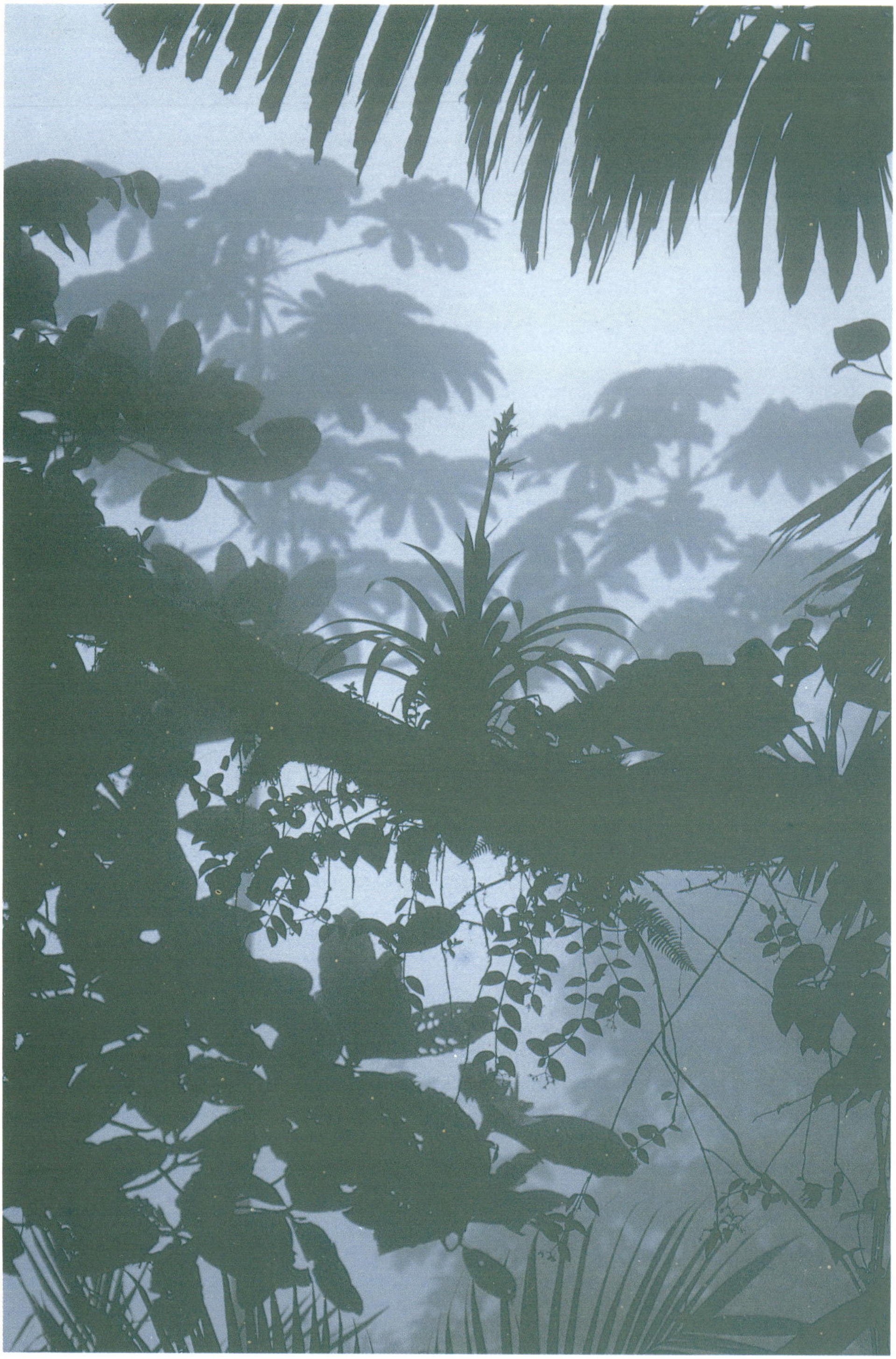

Resting while standing

Despite all your efforts to relax in one of the Zhan Zhuang positions, you may feel that you are becoming tired and tense. Pain in your arms or shoulders may often be the truest signal of the accumulating tension. In that case, you have three possible choices, as outlined below.

1. RELAX AGAIN
First, try again to let your mind go systematically down your body, telling all the points to relax (see p. 44). This is the most beneficial for your entire system – and the method you should aim to develop.

2. REST YOUR HANDS
The second possibility is to reposition your hands so that the backs of your wrists rest in the small of your back, just above your hip bones (see left). Stand like this for a few moments and then resume your Zhan Zhuang standing position. This is an excellent way of relieving the tension in your arms and shoulders, while still allowing a smooth and unobstructed flow of energy through your body. By doing this you will not lose the benefit of the standing exercise. Standing in this position can bring almost instant relief and it is an excellent one to adopt any time in your daily life when you are starting to feel tense and tired.

3. OVERCOME THE BARRIER
The third option when you feel pain and fatigue while training, is to stop. Do this if you feel utterly compelled to and if the previous two measures have had no effect. But beware of stopping only because your nervous system is in temporary revolt. These moments are really the milestones in your training. See if you can cross these barriers and feel the deep, warm comfort that pervades your whole system once you have persevered through your agitation and impatience.

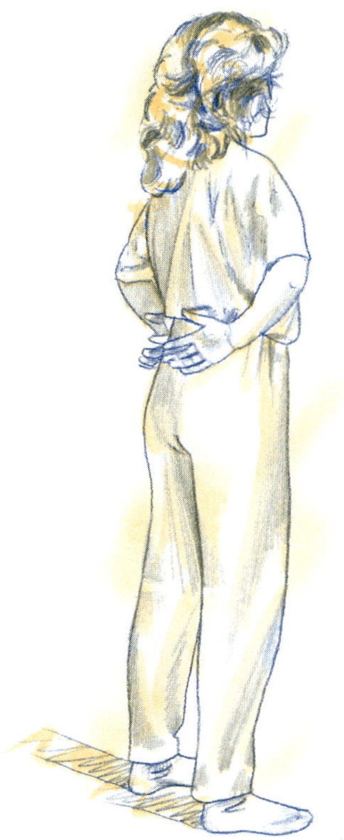

Place the backs of your wrists in the small of your back, just above your hip bones, for a few moments. Then resume your standing position.

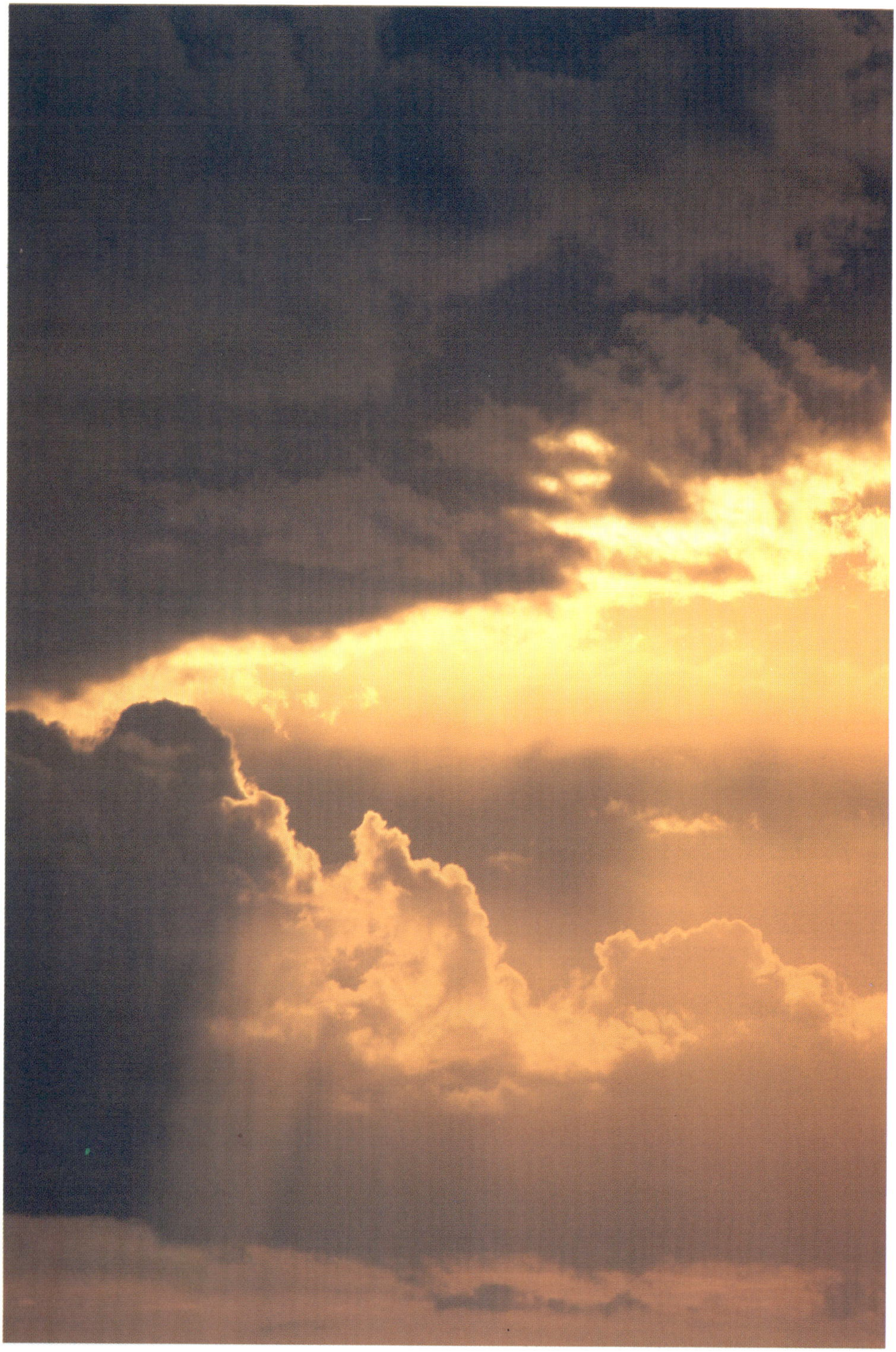

CHAPTER 3
INTERNAL MOVEMENT

Zhan Zhuang training exercises your muscles and your mind. Nothing moves on the outside. The motion is all internal. Some sensations are immediately apparent. You can, for example, feel the muscles in your arms, shoulders, thighs, and calves rapidly reaching the point of exhaustion. As the muscles work harder to hold the position, you can feel your body heat rising. You may begin to sweat and feel your pulse rate speeding up.

If you continue, and force yourself to stand still by a supreme effort of willpower, you will soon be a knot of tension. That tension will cause your muscles to contract further, restricting your blood circulation, and you will run the risk of fainting.

That is not the Way of Energy. At the very point when you start to feel the pain in your muscles, use your mind to tell them to relax (see Chapter 2). This enables oxygen-rich blood to continue to circulate freely through your system at an enhanced rate, rather than being blocked by tense muscles. It also triggers muscle fibres that have not yet been brought into play, and these help carry the load borne by the fibres that are approaching exhaustion. Until you have mastered the art of using your mind to control the tension in your muscles, you can reduce the tension by moving your mind from the pain (see p. 52). Combining this with the correct breathing and relaxation exercises already described in Chapter 2, enables you to hold any of the Zhan Zhuang positions far longer than you could ever imagine to be possible.

The result of all these changes is a high level of internal motion within your body that makes your Chi course through its myriad channels, just as your blood surges through your veins and arteries. Your mental powers are exercised to the full as you learn to control your muscular and nervous systems. Eventually you grow beyond your normal limits of endurance to a highly energized state of alert tranquillity.

The sensations you will experience as you practise the exercises are described in this chapter.

Common sensations

While practising Zhan Zhuang, you will experience a range of sensations in addition to the pain arising from tension. Because we are all different, the sensations we experience will differ. But if you follow the exercise instructions carefully, the work done by your muscles and the resulting activity inside your body is bound to have a strong physical impact. Some people start to sweat a lot; others find parts of the body go cold. Some people tremble and shake; others feel they are going numb. For more than 40 years, Professor Yu Yong Nian (see right) has carefully studied the reactions of well over a thousand students and monitored sensations experienced by beginners. These are all shown on the chart on page 57. This chart helps you to anticipate the sensations you may experience as you begin practising the Zhan Zhuang exercise system. Use it as an encouragement to continue. Bear in mind as you read the chart that no-one follows the reaction pattern precisely: it represents common sensations.

AT THE BEGINNING

Using your mind to relax your muscles may prove very difficult at the beginning. Sometimes the only way you can endure standing for 10 or 20 minutes in the early stages is to take your mind off the pain. You can put on the television or radio, or play some recorded music. This will help to distract you from the pain and thereby reduce the tension that starts to accumulate in your body. You can also talk to anyone who is with you, or sing or daydream, just to take your mind off what you are doing.

TRAINING STAGES

The sensations described in Professor Yu's chart are not limited to the first six weeks of training. They can occur at any point in your training whenever you move to a new level of exercise, such as standing for a longer period of time, adopting a new, advanced posture, or reaching a new mental state.

Note: If you experience no sensations at all, it may be that in your case the exercises take longer to produce these effects. Some people may experience them after only five minutes of standing; others need to stand much longer. The absence of reactions may also stem from the fact that your legs are not bent enough. You may not have sunk down low enough to exceed the normal capacity of your legs to sustain the position. To get the maximum physical benefit from Zhan Zhuang, you need to take yourself gradually beyond your own limits of endurance.

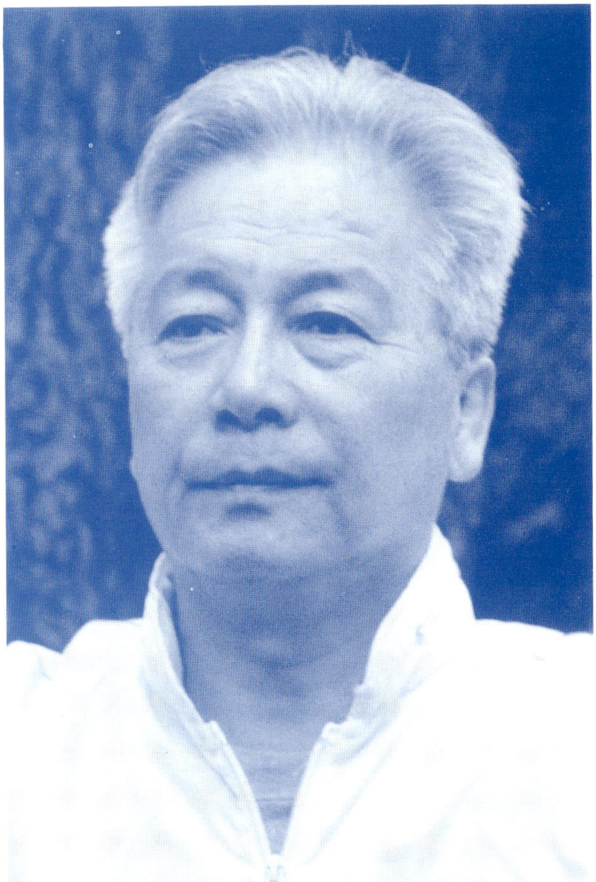

Professor Yu Yong Nian

PROFESSOR YU YONG NIAN

Most mornings in Beijing, you can find Professor Yu Yong Nian in his favourite park teaching Zhan Zhuang. He was born in February 1920 and after completing a training in contemporary Western medicine, and qualifying as a dentist in Japan, he returned to China in 1940. Four years later he started to practise Zhan Zhuang under the personal guidance of Master Wang Xiang Zhai (see p. 58).

In 1953 he began to use aspects of Zhan Zhuang in the treatment of chronic diseases, first at the Beijing Railway Hospital, then in his own health clinic, and later at the Dailin Army Hospital. In 1956, following many successful treatments incorporating the Zhan Zhuang method, he was asked to prepare a report on the medical application of Zhan Zhuang for use in all Chinese hospitals and clinics.

His first book, published (in Chinese) in 1982, has sold about half a million copies. He is an Honorary Member of the Council of the Association of Chi Kung Science of the People's Republic of China and an adviser to the American-Chinese Chi Kung Association.

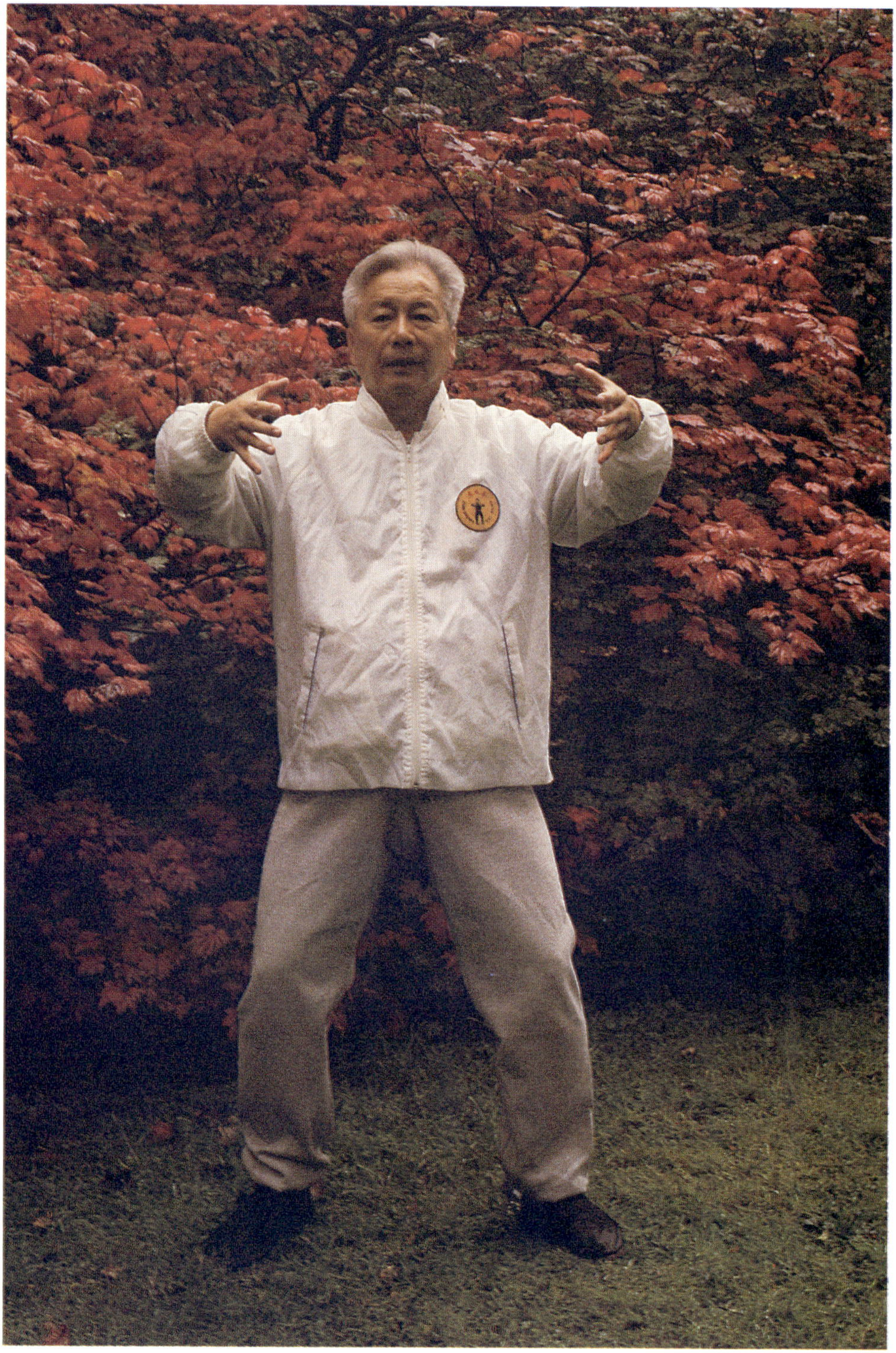

Professor Yu Yong Nian practising Zhan Zhuang.

The chart of Professor Yu Yong Nian

The descriptions that follow and the chart on page 57 will help you understand the signs of internal activity being generated within your organs, muscles, and central nervous system.

NUMBNESS Once you have started Zhan Zhuang training you may feel numbness in some parts of your body while you are performing the standing exercises. This may make you feel very uncomfortable, but it will gradually pass. Different parts may feel numb at different times: you might lose sensation in your hands, head, or feet or in one or both sides of your body. This may then be replaced by (or even start as) a tingling sensation, described by some as feeling like ants walking over your body. You experience these sensations because the pores in your skin are beginning to open, and you can also feel the increased rate of blood circulation at various points under your skin (very often in your fingers and palms at first). These sensations are a result of the increased circulation of your Chi.

ACHING In the first two or three weeks (either after starting at the very beginning or adopting a new posture) you may well experience aches in your legs, knees, ribs, shoulders, or neck. You will probably feel very tired while standing. These are normal reactions. They will pass after a few weeks. If you have old injuries or have had surgery, you may find that the old wounds or scars ache a bit. Similarly, if you suffer from headaches, stomach aches, nervous disorders, digestive problems, or arthritis in your joints, you may find that these manifest themselves while you are standing. This is part of the natural healing and regenerative process unlocked by Zhan Zhuang. The training intensifies the circulation of blood and energy throughout your body, including those regions that have been damaged or blocked off within it. The pain associated with this process normally subsides after about two weeks.

WARMTH Normally, after you adopt any of the positions for 20 minutes, your body temperature rises. Some people begin to sweat profusely, depending on their own make-up and the difficulty of the posture they have adopted. If you reach this point and have begun to sweat, you will probably feel very comfortable afterwards. At the same time, your digestive system will be stimulated and the constant undulating movements of your intestines will be stronger and quicker. This can produce hiccups, burping, flatulence, and stomach rumbling while you are standing. It would be wrong to try to suppress any of this: just let it happen!

SHAKING As you hold the Zhan Zhuang positions your muscles slowly tire. The parts of the muscles that you normally use (working muscles) reach the limits of their endurance and begin to call on the remaining parts of the muscles (resting muscles) to help. This is the point – the stage beyond tension – at which you begin to shake. Often you begin to tremble just a little. But as you persist, the shaking becomes more vigorous and you may end up practically jumping on the spot! Don't worry. Don't try to stop shaking. Just let go and be careful to keep your balance. As you continue to stand, your resting muscles will come into play. You will gradually find yourself shaking less and less until you settle down and are comfortable and at rest. As this happens, it is essential that you concentrate on relaxing. If you can sustain the standing position through this phase and return to quiescent standing, you will have succeeded in taking your body and mind to a higher level of development.

ASYMMETRY While standing, you may feel that one part of your body, which is normally symmetrical with another, has changed in comparison to the other. For example, although you can see that you are holding your hands at the same height, one may feel higher than the other. Or one leg may feel longer than the other. Or one side of your body may react in a different way from the other, by sweating more or by going numb, for example. There can be all sorts of variations: one finger can be hot, another one cold. Usually these sensations disappear after three or four weeks. They may persist for up to three months, but normally not longer than that. Don't worry if you feel these sensations. They are a sign that your training is working.

COMFORT/RELAXATION As you continue with your Zhan Zhuang training, you will begin to feel stronger, more comfortable, and more relaxed as you stand. This is the result of more vigorous blood circulation and the use of your resting muscles. You are absorbing more oxygen, your mind and central nervous system are relaxed but alert, and your natural energy is flowing in an increasingly unimpeded way through your system. The goal is to make this a daily experience.

The first column of the chart (opposite) lists the general sensations most commonly experienced by people in the first six weeks of Zhan Zhuang training: numbness; aching; warmth; shaking; asymmetry, and comfort/relaxation. The more precise reactions in each of these categories are listed in the next column. For example, beside the general sensation of "asymmetry" are listed six specific reactions where one side of the body or one limb begins to feel different (longer, higher, hotter) than the other limb or side of the body. Over the columns indicating the six weeks, the possible degree of each reaction is indicated by plus and minus signs. Your own experience may not correspond exactly to this.

The chart of Professor Yu Yong Nian

General sensation	Specific reaction	WEEK1	WEEK2	WEEK3	WEEK4	WEEK5	WEEK6
NUMBNESS	Hands numb	+	+	++	++	+	–
	Feet numb	+	+	++	++	+	–
	Head numb	–	–	–	±	±	±
	One side of the body numb	–	–	–	±	±	±
	Whole body numb	–	–	–	–	±	±
	Tingling (ants on body)	–	±	±	±	+	+
ACHING	Aching shoulder	+	++	+	±	–	–
	Aching neck	–	–	+	++	+	–
	Aching knee	+	++	++	+	±	–
	Aching leg	+	++	+	–	–	–
	Aching hip and ribs	–	±	±	–	–	–
	Pain in old injuries	–	±	+	–	–	–
	Increased pain in current ailments	–	–	±	+	–	–
WARMTH	Hiccuping/burping	±	+	+	+	±	±
	Flatulence	±	+	+	+	±	±
	Rumbling stomach	–	–	–	±	±	±
	Rising body heat	±	+	+	+	–	–
	Sweating	±	+	+	+	±	–
SHAKING	Trembling	–	+	+	+	–	–
	Strong shaking	–	–	+	+	–	–
	Jumping	–	–	–	+	+	–
ASYMMETRY	One hand feels higher than the other	+	+	+	+	+	+
	One leg feels longer than the other	–	–	+	+	+	+
	One hand, leg, or side feels numb	–	–	–	±	±	±
	One side of the body sweats	–	–	±	±	+	+
	Blood circulation feels faster in one side of the body	–	–	–	±	+	+
	Body temperature feels different on each side	–	–	±	±	+	+
COMFORT/ RELAXATION	Head	–	–	+	+	++	+++
	Chest	–	–	+	+	++	+++
	Whole body	–	–	+	+	++	+++

KEY

– no sensation
± minor sensation
+ sensation occurs
++ strong sensation
+++ intense feeling

"What does your father teach you?"

My master, Professor Yu Yong Nian, studied dentistry in Japan. When he returned to China after his studies he was exhausted and far from fit. His friends told him: do some exercise like Tai Chi Chuan. But it left him breathless. He thought: if I am so lacking in energy, how will I be able to put in long, hard hours as a dentist?

Someone told him that a new system of energy training had been developed: Zhan Zhuang. He was ready to try anything and went to see Master Wang Xiang Zhai who was teaching in a Beijing park. Like all beginners he was told just to stand still, like a tree. He stood there absolutely still, but all around him in the class he could see older students practising vigorous fighting movements. He thought to himself: why am I being treated so badly? Why am I being made to stand like this? Does the master think I'm lazy?

He was so convinced that he was being denied the teaching he was after, that he befriended the Master's son in the hope of finding out what was going on. Finally he asked him: "What does your father teach you?", thinking that he would find out the highest secrets of the art. "Oh," said Master Wang's son, "He teaches me to stand like a tree." Amazed, Yu asked him: "Does he tell you why you must do this?" "Oh no," came the immediate reply, "He just tells me to stand like this every day and if I don't he beats me."

After giving this strange new exercise a try, Yu gave up and just concentrated on his work. But he soon noticed his energy declining. He looked back to the first few months when he had stood like a tree in the park, and realized how much fitter he had felt then. So he returned to Master Wang.

One day, three years later, Master Wang asked him to fight one of his other students, a labourer who had put in years of practice in the martial arts. Young Yu was taken aback. He had no fighting experience. But Master Wang insisted. The two began to grapple with each other and much to Yu's amazement he found that he could easily control and overpower his experienced opponent. He suddenly realized he had a power within him that he had never used.

From that time onward his study deepened and he eventually reached the honoured position of working closely with Master Wang to develop the Zhan Zhuang system and its use for health and healing.

After Master Wang's death, Yu's work and study continued and now, in his seventies, he still teaches in Beijing Park. In 1989 he published his fourth book on Zhan Zhuang, a small instruction manual with the results of his research (in Chinese). It was completely sold out within a week.

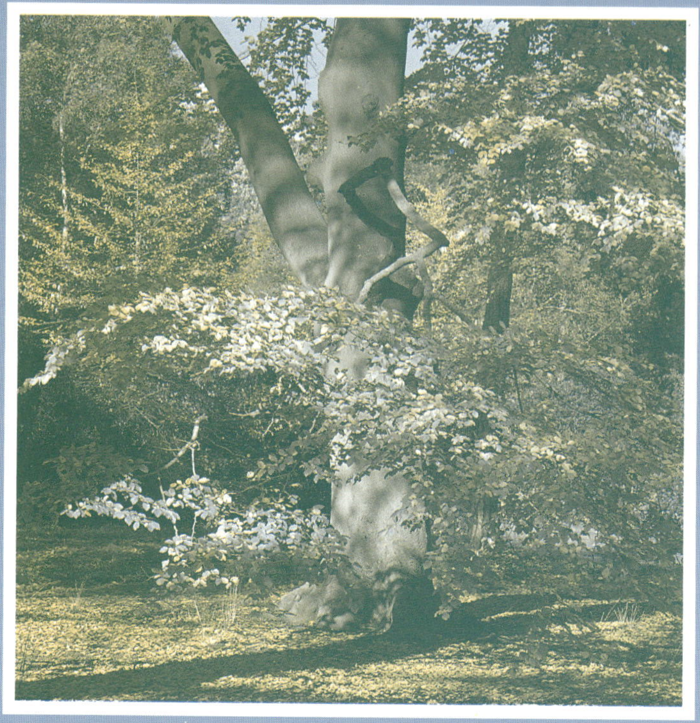

PART TWO

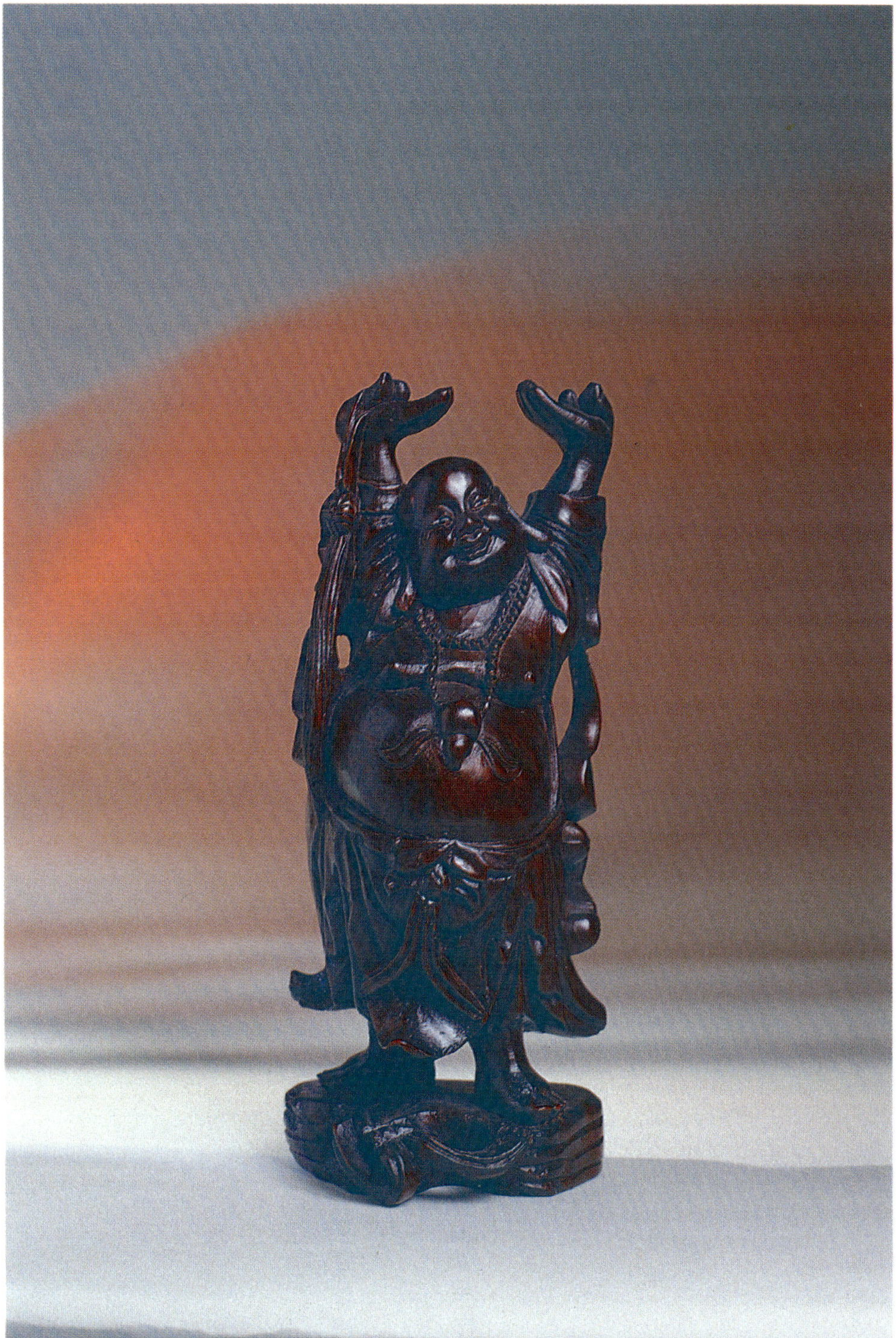

The Buddha performs Ba Duan Jin.

CHAPTER 4
PREPARING FOR ENERGY

After you have practised the first two standing exercises of Zhan Zhuang for several months, you will notice that important changes will have started taking place in your body. Some of the blockages in the pathways of your internal energy will have been cleared. As you stand, you will begin to feel the unusual sensations of trembling and tingling as explained in Chapter 3. Your oxygen-enriched blood and Chi will be flowing faster and more vigorously throughout your system.

You are ready to move on to the next stage of your development. Since you will be generating much higher levels of energy than your body has previously been accustomed to, you need to strengthen the capacity of your system to handle and transport the new flow of power.

The ancient Chinese developed a unique set of exercises precisely for toning up the internal organs and systems. It is still practised to this day by Chinese people all over the world. It is known as Ba Duan Jin, literally translated as "Eight Strands of Brocade" and sometimes called the "Eight Fine Exercises". The exercises develop the most important systems of the body, yet can be safely practised by almost anyone of any age without fear of strain or injury.

The description of the benefits that each of the following exercises brings may seem odd. For example, it is not obvious how stretching your hands upward to the sky affects your heart and kidneys. The answer lies in the network of Chi channels (meridians) identified by Chinese medicine in the human body (see pp. 18). These are connected to your vital organs but they also run through your body as far as your fingertips and toes. Each of the Ba Duan Jin exercises intensifies the flow of energy along the full length of specific meridians and thus the complete set of exercises benefits the whole network, including the internal organs through which that energy passes. Regular practice is the ideal preparation you need to carry the "awakened dragon" of your Chi.

Starting Ba Duan Jin

Once you begin these exercises, you should make every effort to do them regularly – and to do the full set of eight. Just a few minutes every day will be sufficient. This is the way to get the full benefit from them. Their natural life-enhancing effect will not be nearly as pronounced if you do them in bursts for a few days and then do nothing for a week or two.

Once you have learned the eight exercises, and are smoothly stretching into all the positions, you can move on to the more advanced positions shown for each exercise. These will increase the stretch and intensify the flow of Chi.

WHEN AND WHERE TO PRACTISE

The ideal time to practise is in the morning, as the regular prelude to any of the standing exercises. If this is not possible, you can do these exercises later in the day, always leaving at least an hour after eating. If you do them on a full stomach, you might adversely affect your breathing and digestion. Some people do them before sleeping. This is fine, but still remember to allow an hour after dinner.

Always try to practise where the air is fresh. The Chinese way is to exercise out of doors. But if this is not possible for you or the weather is inclement, then use a well-ventilated room.

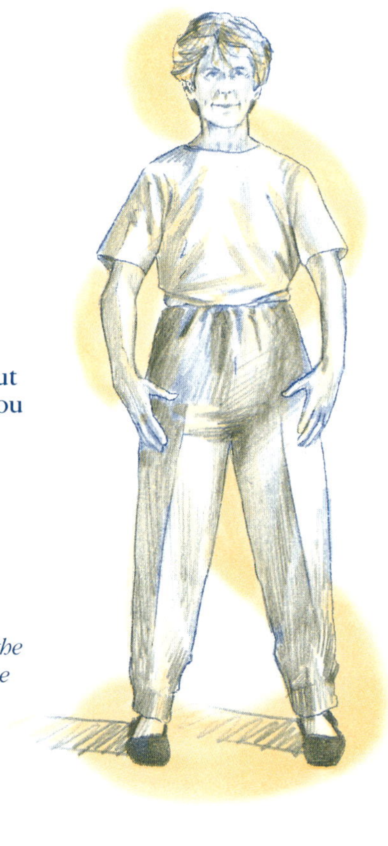

Standing in the Wu Chi – the opening position for all the Ba Duan Jin exercises.

Before you begin

STRETCH AND RELAX
Begin slowly and gently. Relax your muscles and nerves – there is no benefit from tension. Stretch carefully and thoroughly, paying full attention to the correct positions and to the advice given with each exercise.

IMMEDIATE SENSATIONS
You are likely to feel the natural warmth of your body increasing as you go through the eight exercises. You may perspire slightly. But do not expect to be left exhausted, with strained muscles, sweating profusely, and gasping for breath. This is a powerful system of exercise, but it is not meant to be a set of physical jerks! Ba Duan Jin is based on a completely different philosophy of health and personal growth. It emphasizes the careful development of all the body's vital systems and aims to care for you at whatever age and level of fitness you have reached, rather than impose unbearable strains on you.

BREATHE NATURALLY
Breathe calmly through your nose, keeping your mouth gently closed. Don't try to alter the rate of your natural breathing. Don't try to breathe more deeply or slowly. Your breathing will become fuller over time as your capacity grows. You will begin to develop natural abdominal breathing (see pp. 42-43), easing and increasing the rhythmic movement of your diaphragm. This, in turn, will have a wonderful effect on all the organs in your abdominal cavity as they begin to benefit from regular, internal massage.

You must let this process mature naturally within you. Don't interfere with it by forcing the pace. Just let every breath come and go in its own way.

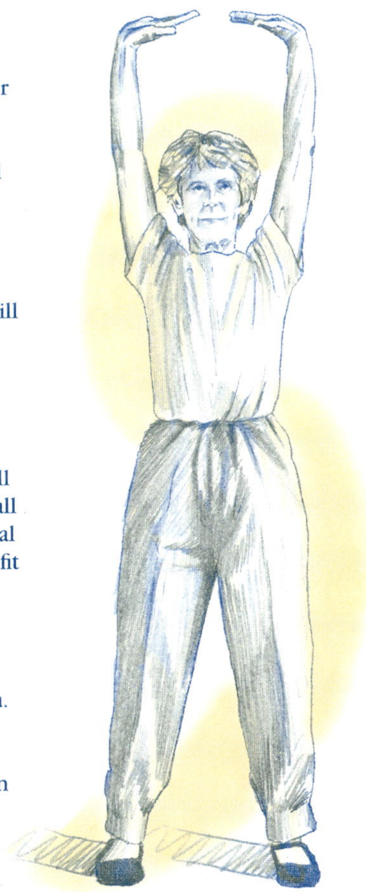

Supporting the Sky with Both Hands – advanced position (see p. 67).

1. Supporting the Sky with Both Hands Regulates All Internal Organs

This opening exercise regulates all internal organs, from your heart and lungs in your upper torso through to your kidneys and intestines in your lower abdomen. It relieves fatigue, increases inhalation, and helps prepare your body for the exercises that follow. It also helps invigorate the muscles and bones of your back and waist and can help correct poor posture of the upper back and shoulders.

STARTING THE EXERCISE

Start in the Wu Chi position: feet a shoulder-width apart, shoulders relaxed, arms hanging loosely at your sides (see p. 64). Face straight ahead. Then slowly raise your arms, keeping your shoulders relaxed, as if you were lifting an invisible balloon in front of you. As you raise your arms, breathe in.

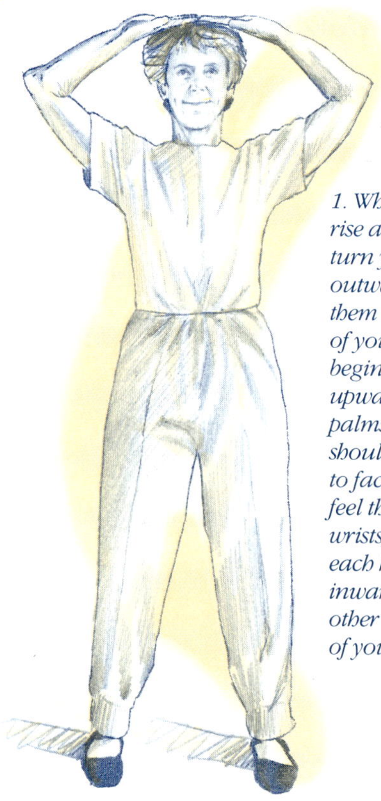

1. When your hands rise above your head, turn your palms outward and bring them above the crown of your head, ready to begin pressing straight upward. Your flat palms and fingers should be fully turned to face the sky (you will feel the stretch in your wrists). The fingers of each hand should face inward toward each other over the middle of your head.

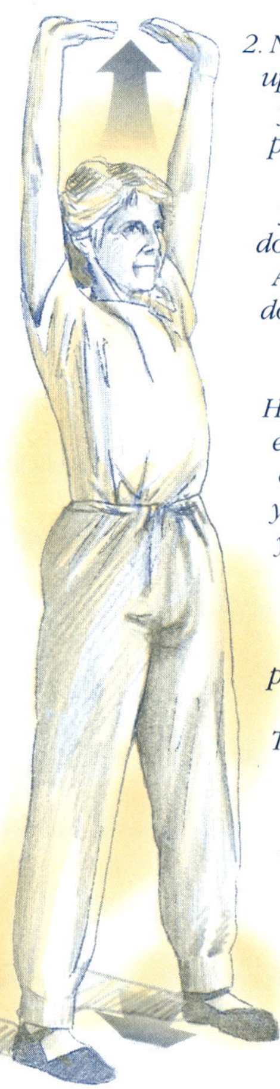

2. Now press both hands upward, straightening your arms as fully as possible – your hands need not touch. Let your feet press firmly down into the ground. As you stretch up and down simultaneously, breathe out.

Hold your arms in the extended position for one second. Then, as you breathe in, lower your arms so that the backs of your hands are just above your head, and ease the pressure on your feet. Pause for a second. Then repeat the cycle, moving your hands up and down over your head until you have done this eight times.

THE NEXT STAGE
When you feel that you have mastered the smoothly stretching arm motions, with your hands in the correct positions, and when you can synchronize the extending and contracting movements of your arms with the gentle inhalation and exhalation of your breath, you can take the exercise to the next stage.

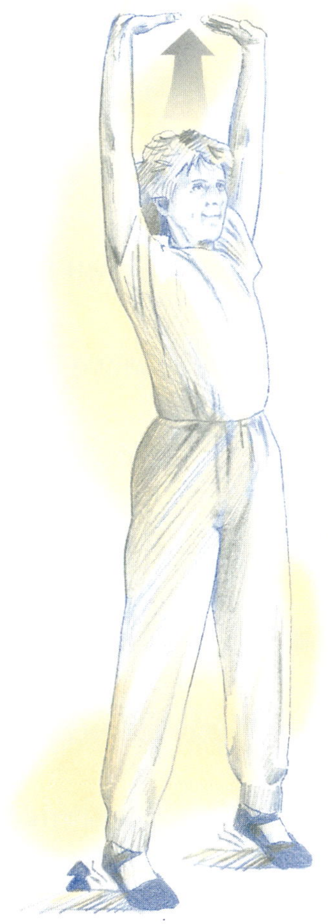

3. As you begin to press upward with your hands, slowly rise up on your toes so that you complete the full extension of your arms and legs at the same time. This is also excellent for developing your sense of balance.

Advanced level

After at least a year of regular practice, you can advance to the next stage of this exercise. Extend your hands above your head, palms facing upward as in the basic level. Keep your feet flat on the floor. Now imagine that you are pushing against a heavy stone block above your head. Breathe out as you imagine you are using about 20 per cent of your strength to press upward against the stone and downward into the ground. Then, instead of lowering your arms when you have finished exhaling, relax, keeping your arms and hands still extended, and breathe in. Then imagine trying to move the block again as you breathe out, this time using 40 per cent of your power. Relax again, breathe in, keeping your hands in position, and then repeat a further six times, imagining that you are progressively increasing the pressure in both directions. Go up, gradually increasing your power, to 50, 60, 70, 80, 90, and – on the eighth exhalation – finally to 100 per cent.

2. Drawing a Bow to Each Side Resembles Shooting an Eagle

This exercise places the emphasis on your thorax – the home of your heart and lungs – thus greatly improving the circulation of blood and oxygen. It also improves the flow of energy in your small intestine.

STARTING THE EXERCISE
Starting in the Wu Chi position, unlock your knees (see p. 64). Then gently raise your hands so that they face your chest. Imagine that you are holding an invisible balloon between your arms and your chest.

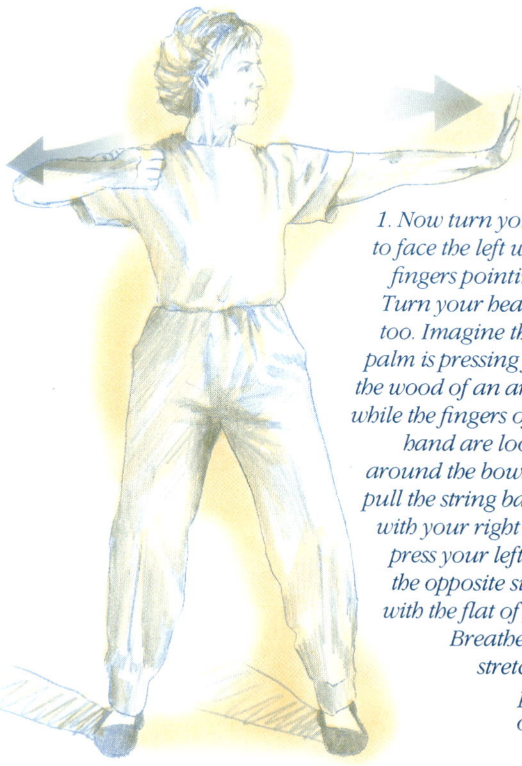

1. Now turn your left palm to face the left with all your fingers pointing upward. Turn your head to the left, too. Imagine that your left palm is pressing flat against the wood of an archer's bow, while the fingers of your right hand are loosely curled around the bowstring. Now pull the string back, leading with your right elbow, and press your left arm out to the opposite side, leading with the flat of your hand. Breathe out as you stretch. Hold the position for one second.

2. Then, while breathing in, slowly bring your arms back round to the front of your chest. Repeat the exercise to the right side. Complete a total of eight drawings of the bow, four to each side, alternately.

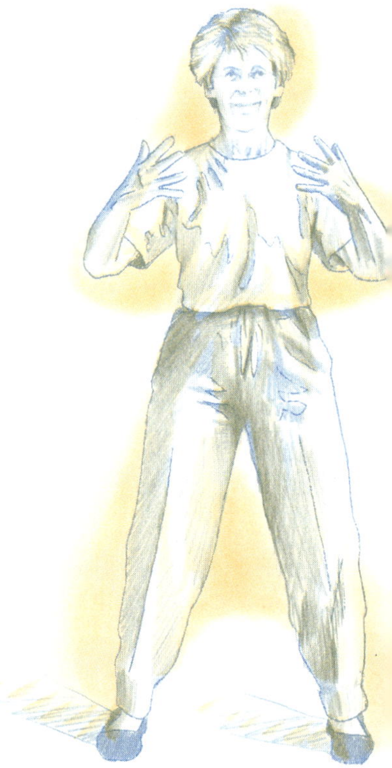

THE NEXT STAGE
When you are comfortable with the movements and getting over the stiffness of your wrists (you will probably find it difficult at first to keep your palm and fingers constantly at a right-angle to your arm throughout the stretch), you can go on to the next level.

3. Straighten your legs. Raise only the index finger of your "bow" hand, leaving the others loosely curled. Try to push your palm and index finger up at right-angles to your arm throughout the stretch (see below).

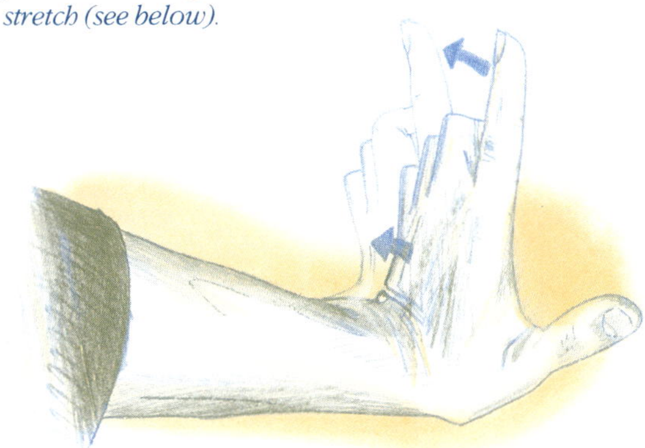

INCREASED CHI
Don't worry if you feel pain, stiffness, or strange sensations in your finger as you do this. Just keep trying to straighten it up. As you advance you may feel it "buzzing", or "tingling", or vibrating inside – a sure sign of the increased flow of Chi.

Advanced level

You can advance to the next stages of this exercise after one or two years of regular practice. Imagine that you are in control of two bows, one running down either side of your spine. This time the strings are controlled by your hands with the index fingers erect. Push both bowstrings simultaneously, keeping the palms and index fingers of both hands upright at 90 degrees to your arms. Do this eight times in all, breathing out each time you push the two bows, and then breathing in as you allow your hands to come back toward your torso and relax.

A further stage of this advanced exercise is to extend your arms to either side of your body and to bring your mind into play. Your palms and all fingers point up at right-angles to your arms. Imagine that your palms and fingers are pressing outward against two flat slabs of stone. Breathe out as you apply 20 per cent of your pressure in both directions. Then relax and breathe in, but keep your arms extended in place. As you exhale, imagine pressing the slabs again. Each time imagine that you are using increased pressure in both directions, eight times in all – 40, 50, 60, 70, 80, 90, and 100 per cent.

Finally, bring your arms back toward the middle of your body as you inhale. Lower them as you exhale.

3. Holding Up a Single Hand Regulates the Spleen and Stomach

The movements of this exercise increase the flow of energy along both sides of your body, and benefit your liver, gall bladder, spleen, and stomach. They help to prevent diseases of the gastro-intestinal tract.

STARTING THE EXERCISE
Begin by raising your hands from the Wu Chi position (see p. 64) so that you hold an invisible balloon between them. Then turn your right palm upward and your left palm downward.

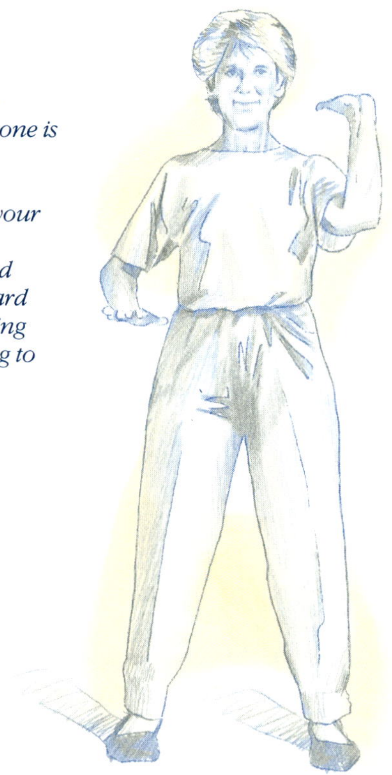

1. Now extend your two hands so that your right one is poised above your right shoulder, palm facing upward, turned so that your fingers are pointing backward. Your left hand extends downward toward your left thigh, palm facing the floor, fingers pointing to the front.

2. Now straighten your arms, pressing both hands apart at the same time – the right upward and the left downward – keeping the palms flat and at right-angles to your arms. Move your two arms so that they extend fully at the same time. Breathe out as your arms move apart and press upward and downward. Hold for one second.

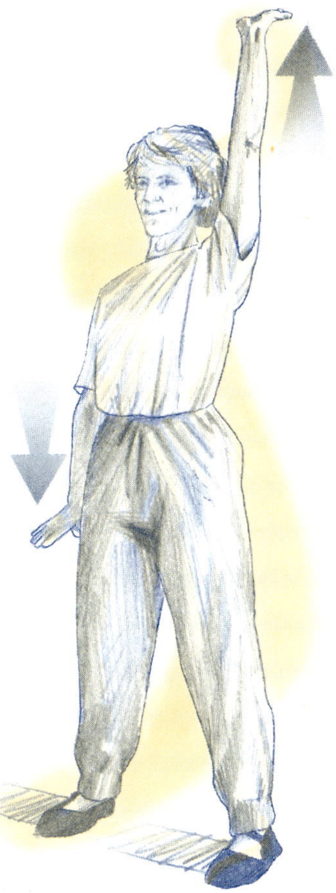

COMPLETING THE EXERCISE

Relax and breathe in as you bring both hands back in front of your body, both palms turned gently upward, as if you were carrying something in front of you.

Then turn your palms and repeat the exercise in the opposite directions, left hand moving up and right hand moving down, as you exhale. Complete four full cycles of both movements – eight extensions of the arms in all.

Advanced level

After regular practice of the basic level of this exercise for about a year, you can advance to the next level.

After you extend your palms fully (see step 2, above), leave your hands in that position, breathe out, and imagine that you are using 20 per cent of your power to press apart two huge blocks of stone. As you do so, twist slightly to the side with your hand facing down, and breathe out. Keeping your hands in place, relax and breathe in. Then, on the next breath out, imagine pressing the blocks apart with 40 per cent of your strength and twist a little further to the side, as if you were turning like a screw. Then, without moving, relax and breathe in.

Continue the exercise increasing your twist each time using 50, 60, 70, 80, 90, and 100 per cent of your power each time you breathe out, increasing your twist each time until you are turned fully to the side. After that, slowly unwind as you breathe in. Change sides and repeat.

4. Looking Back Like a Cow Gazing at the Moon

This is one of the most potent of the eight exercises. It has a powerful effect on your central nervous system and the circulation of both blood and Chi to your head. It stimulates the vital power of your kidneys. It also strengthens the activity of your eyeballs, your neck and shoulder muscles, and your nerves, and is excellent for alleviating high blood pressure and hardening of the arteries.
CAUTION Do not practise this Ba Duan Jin exercise when pregnant.

STARTING THE EXERCISE
Begin by lifting your arms from the Wu Chi position (see p. 64) so that you hold a large imaginary balloon between your arms and your chest.

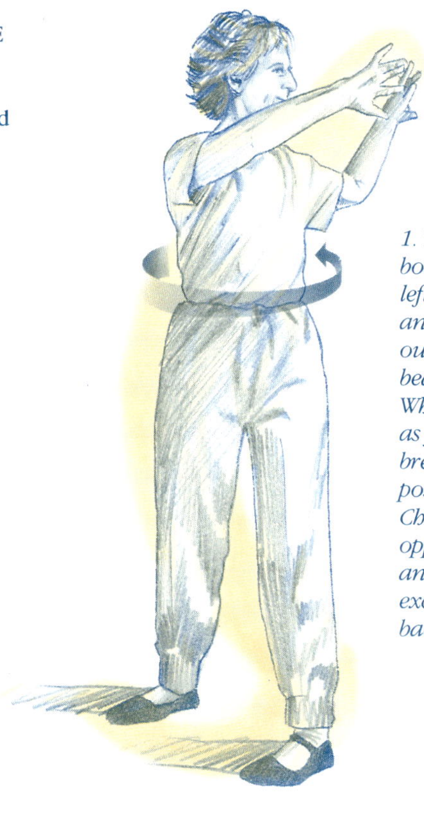

1. Turn your entire upper body from your hips, to the left. Breathe out as you move, and turn your palms outward as if pushing a large beach ball away from you. When you have turned as far as your hips will allow, finish breathing out and hold the position for one second. Check that your hands are still opposite the front of your chest and not skewed sideways by excessive twisting of your upper back and shoulders.

2. Turn back toward the front as you breathe in. As you move, turn your hands back inward to their original position, embracing the invisible balloon between your arms and chest. Relax and stay in this position for one second and finish breathing in.

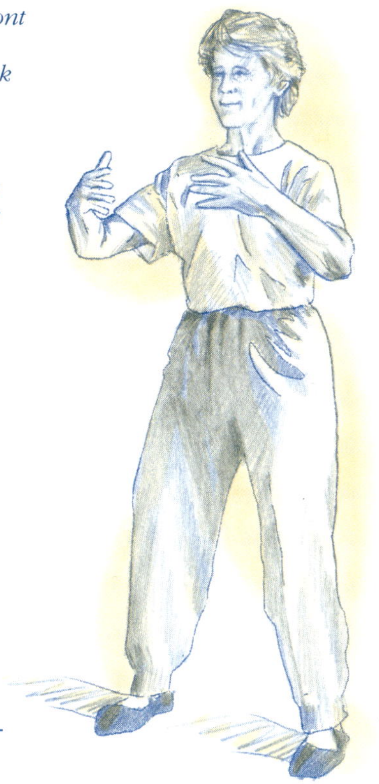

COMPLETING THE EXERCISE
Turn to the right, performing the same twist. Do this exercise four times to each side alternately.

Be sure to keep both feet flat on the floor throughout. This is essential to help draw the energy of the earth in through your feet as you do this exercise. Many of the vital energy meridians in your body stretch to your feet or have their origins there and it is essential to keep the contact from the soles of your feet and the ends of your toes right up through your back, neck, palms, and fingers.

Advanced level

Practise this exercise regularly at the basic level for one or two years and then advance to the next stage.

When you turn to the left, imagine that your hands are pressing against an enormous ball of stone. As you breathe out imagine that you are pressing up from the floor and through your hands, initially with 20 per cent of your strength. Hold the position for one second.

Then, keeping your hands in place, breathe in and relax. This will cause your whole body to turn naturally ever so slightly back toward the front. Allow this to happen and finish breathing in.

Then, as you breathe out again, twist from your hips a little further to the side and imagine that you are using 40 per cent of your strength to press against the stone ball. Hold for one second, then relax and allow the slight natural recoil of your body to take place.

Repeat on the same side, progressively using 50, 60, 70, 80, 90, and ultimately 100 per cent of your power each time you twist and breathe out.

Then perform the same sequence to the other side.

5. Lowering the Head and Hips Removes Excess Heat from the Heart

The explanations for the value of this exercise include prevention against fever and reduction of tension in the sympathetic nervous system. It certainly has a powerful relaxing effect and, as such, eases the flow of energy along a number of your body's meridians.

CAUTION Do not practise this Ba Duan Jin exercise when pregnant.

1. From the Wu Chi position (see p. 64), raise your right hand in an arc over your head with your hand held palm downward.

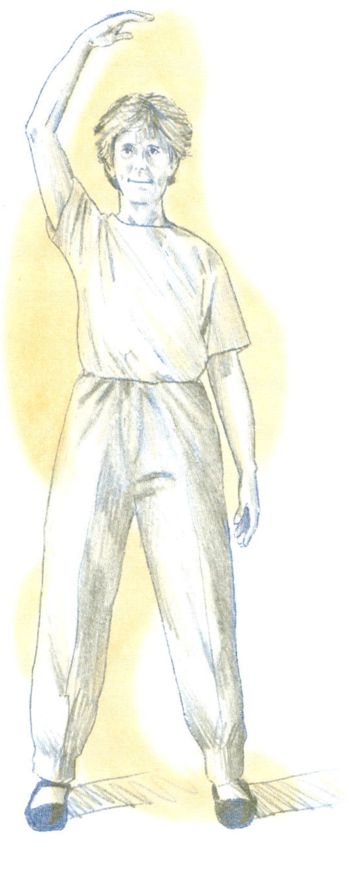

2. Breathe out as you bend over to your left. Keep your right arm curved above your head, letting your left arm hang naturally down by your side. Transfer all your weight to your right leg, allowing your left heel to rise slightly off the ground. Your body will arc outward naturally to the right, with both hands sinking loosely downward to the left. Stay there for one second. Stay relaxed.

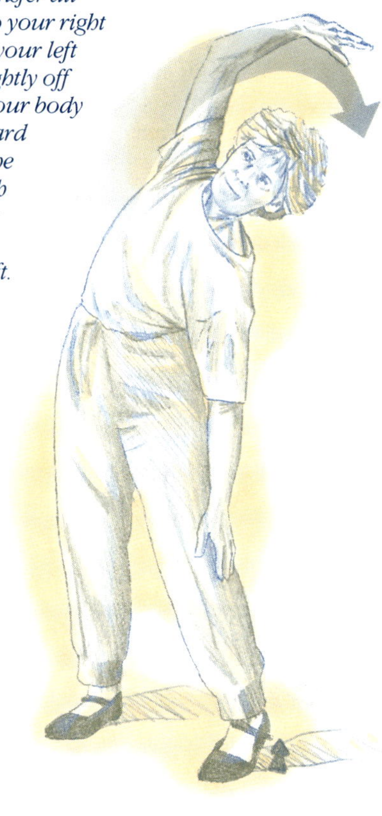

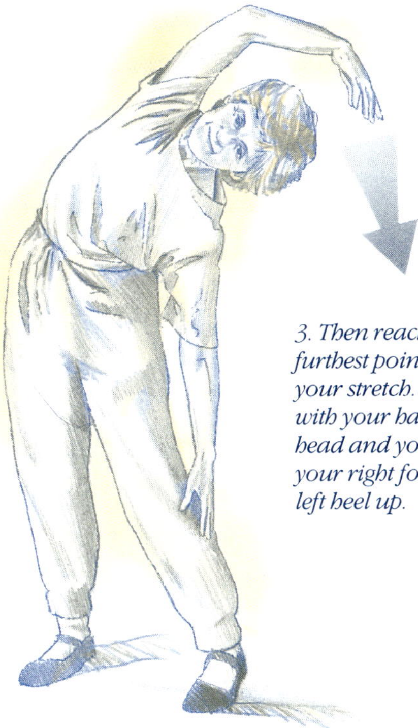

3. Then reach over to the furthest point of comfort in your stretch. Hold the position with your hand over your head and your weight still on your right foot, keeping your left heel up.

COMPLETING THE EXERCISE
Breathe in as you come up and repeat to the right side. Complete four stretches to each side alternately.

Advanced level

After you have practised these stretches for a year or two, you can progress to the advanced levels.

First, instead of transferring your weight to the outer leg of the arc of your stretch, do the opposite. For example, when you bend over to the left, transfer your full weight to your left leg. Keep it straight as you bend over on that side, and allow your right heel to lift slightly off the ground. Do this for the sequence of eight stretches.

After practising the exercise in this new way for about a year – to increase the stretch and adjust your sense of balance – you can advance to a further level.

As you breathe out and bend over to the left, imagine a magnetic current running between your left foot (which is flat on the floor, bearing all your weight) and your two hands (which are forming an arc toward the ground). Imagine the magnetic force is pulling with 20 per cent of its strength. Finish breathing out. Stay relaxed, without changing position, and take a small breath.

Breathe out again, this time imagining the force has increased to 40 per cent of its strength, pulling your hands closer to the ground. Then relax and breathe in, staying in that position. Complete eight pulls on that side, and progressively increase the power of the magnet to 100 per cent of its strength.

Then straighten up and repeat the same exercise stretching to the right side.

6. Touching the Feet with Both Hands Reinforces the Kidneys and Loins

This exercise is good for the muscles of your lower back and legs and for stretching your spine. It is also beneficial for the internal organs of your lower abdomen. The movements of your waist actually bring every tissue and organ of your abdomen into play. The whole exercise strengthens your kidneys, your adrenal glands, and the arteries, veins, and nerves associated with them. Since your kidneys play a vital role in regulating the water metabolism of your entire body, this exercise helps maintain a healthy balance in your internal environment.
CAUTION Do not practise this Ba Duan Jin exercise when pregnant.

1. Starting in the Wu Chi position (see p. 64), raise your arms out to the sides to shoulder height.

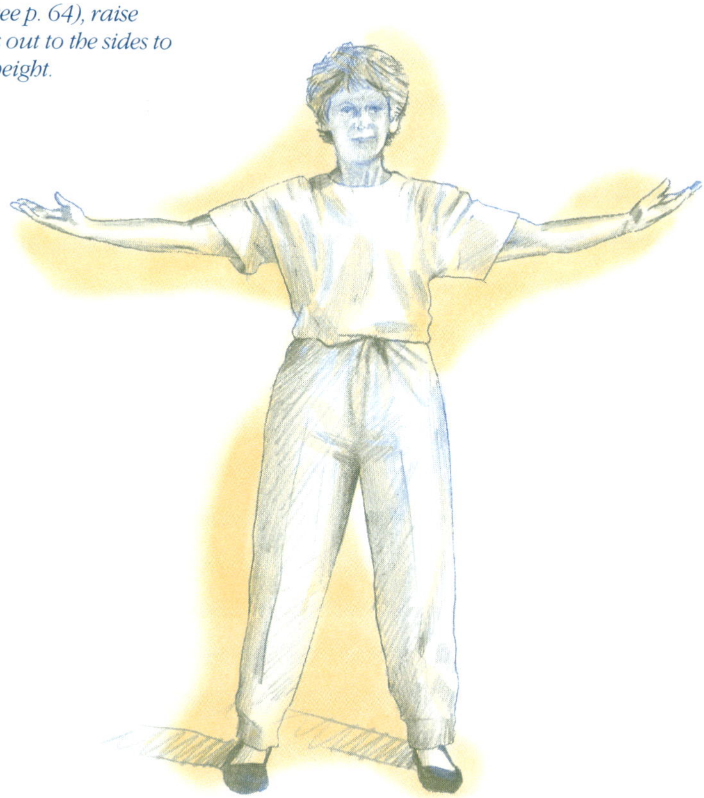

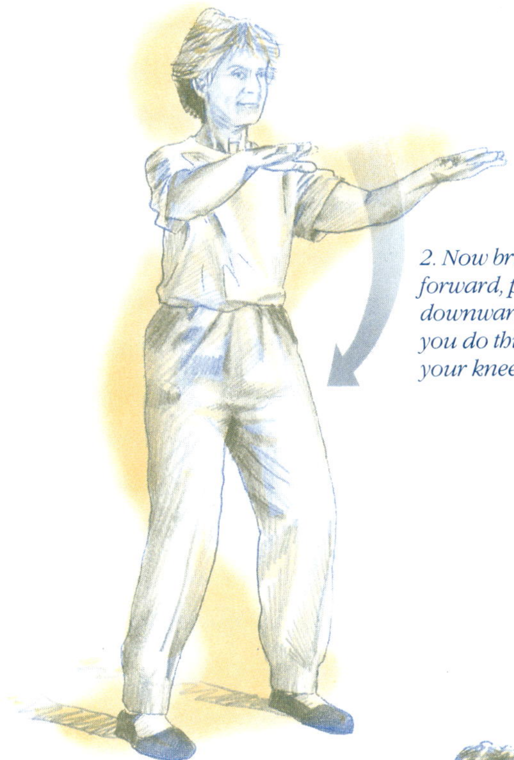

2. *Now bring your arms forward, palms facing downward. Breathe in as you do this. Begin to bend your knees slightly.*

Advanced level

After a year or so of regular practice, you can move on to the next level.

Keeping your feet flat on the ground, lower yourself to a full squat. Remember to breathe out completely as you go down. This time your hands should brush over your toes as they circle down and around. Your circling arms will also help your balance. Look straight ahead. Try to keep your back vertical but not stiff. Don't crouch too far forward, but don't stiffen up so much that you lose your balance and fall backward. Resist the temptation to speed up; try to do this exercise calmly, slowly, and smoothly.

3. *Continue to bend at the knees, lowering yourself halfway down as if beginning a full squat position. Breathe out as you go down, and circle your arms down in front of you. When you reach the half squat position, hold it for one second. Imagine that you are resting your bottom on a very large, inflated balloon. Your hands will have come down to a point roughly level with your hips.*

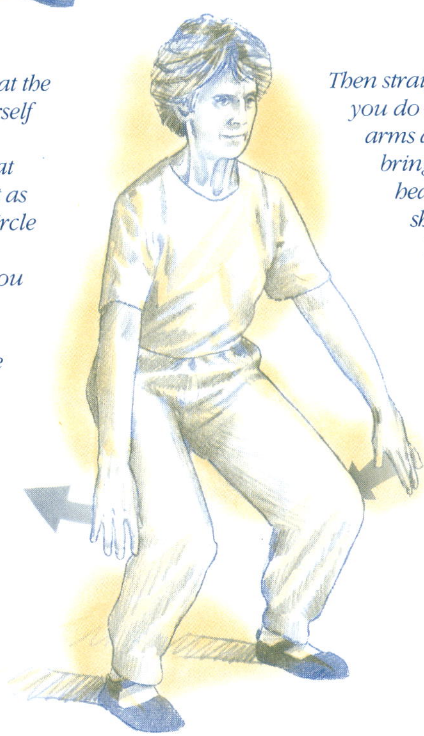

Then straighten up as you breathe in. As you do this, continue circling your arms around behind you (see left), bringing them up and over your head to rest in front of you at shoulder height where they began. Your hands should finish in this position by the time you are standing up.

Make eight full circles, moving slowly and steadily, letting your arms drop down as far as you can at the lowest point of the circles.

7. Clenching the Fists Increases Strength

This exercise develops the flow of Chi from your feet through your entire body and extends it through your hands and eyes. It excites your cerebral cortex and related nerves, and speeds the circulation of blood and oxygen in your cardiovascular system. This is not a punching exercise – it is designed to strengthen the flow of your internal power: it must be done slowly and calmly with great concentration. Each movement begins gently and the full power comes in only at the end of each extension.
CAUTION Do not practise this Ba Duan Jin exercise when pregnant.

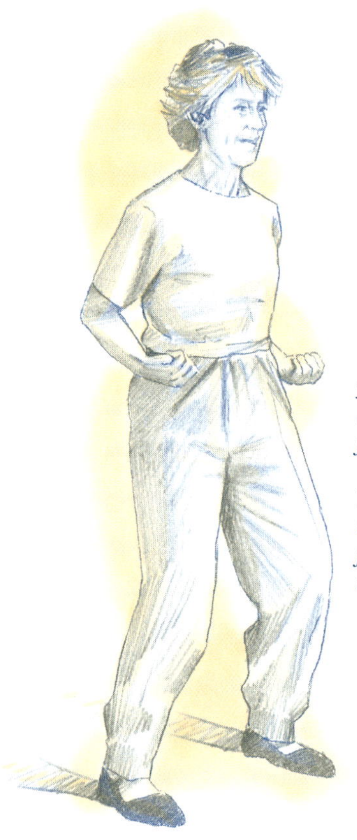

STARTING THE EXERCISE
Standing in the Wu Chi position (see p. 64), slightly bend your knees.

1. Fold your thumbs inside your fists (see right) and hold them beside your hips, palms facing upward. Breathe in.

You may find it uncomfortable to hold your thumb inside your fist at first, but as you persevere it will become easier.

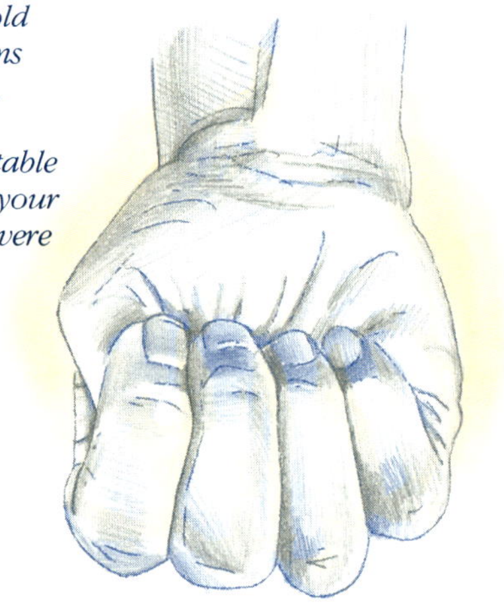

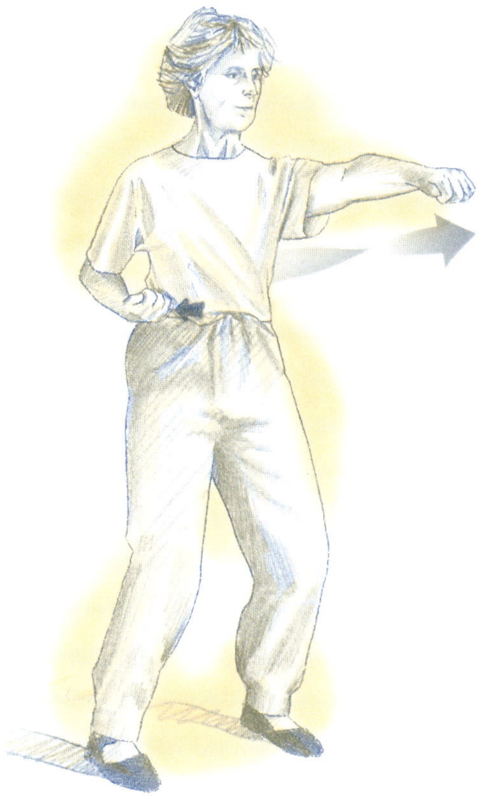

2. As you breathe out, extend your left arm slowly forward at chest height, turning your fist over to finish palm down. At the same time, pull your right elbow back beside you. Look straight ahead and hold the position for one second.

Repeat the exercise eight times, alternately extending your left and right arms.

Advanced level

Practise this level after a year or two of performing the basic exercise.

Start facing straight ahead, with your feet flat on the floor and your toes pointing forward. Then twist about 45 degrees to the left, without moving your feet.

Begin to extend your arms as in the basic exercise. Your fists will still move straight out from your shoulders, but will be directed naturally toward the left.

As you extend your arms, it is very important at the advanced level to do the following four things at the same time.

First, breathe out fully through your nose.

Second, squeeze the fingers of both fists around the thumbs – so that your thumbs are pressed tightly toward your palms.

Third, clench your teeth tightly.

Fourth, open your eyes as wide as you can and glare intently straight ahead.

The combination of these four movements greatly strengthens the power of this exercise.

8. Shaking the Body Wards off All Illnesses

This exercise aims to refresh and regenerate all your internal organs by enabling them to massage each other. It is also excellent for your spine, your nervous system, and your sense of balance.

CAUTION Do not practise this Ba Duan Jin exercise when pregnant.

STARTING THE EXERCISE

Standing in the Wu Chi position (see p. 64), lower yourself slightly by bending your knees.

Rest the backs of your hands on the flesh just above your hip bones on either side of your lower back. Shake your whole body by bouncing gently up and down from your knees. Your feet stay flat on the ground. Make sure your shoulders and elbows are completely relaxed so that their weight rests on the backs of your hands. You will feel your hands pleasantly massaging your lower back.

On each bounce, breathe out through your nose in little bursts, until you have exhaled completely. Keep bouncing as you inhale smoothly. Continue until you have completed eight exhalations and inhalations.

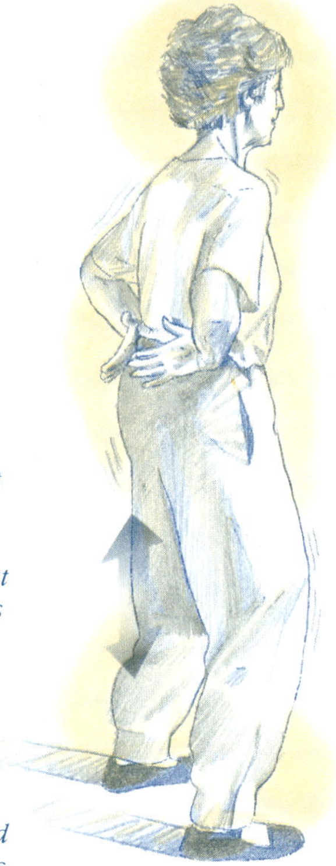

Advanced level

Although there is an advanced level for this exercise, it is not included in this book since there is a slight risk that some people might injure themselves if they attempt it without the guidance of an instructor. However, the benefit of the basic level of the exercise is considerable and it can be practised in combination with the advanced levels of the other exercises without causing any problem.

The Buddha performs Ba Duan Jin

If you go into a Chinese arts and crafts shop, take a look at the rows of little statues and porcelain figurines. You will find the traditional gods of happiness and good fortune. You will almost certainly find the beautiful goddess of mercy and compassion, Kwan Yin. Among the many figures you may also come across a smiling Buddha with a little fat belly (see the photograph on page 62). He is standing up with his arms stretched over his head. His palms press against the sky and his fingers face inward to meet over his head. He is performing the opening exercise of Ba Duan Jin, as anybody acquainted with these matters will instantly recognize.

Like all popular traditions in any culture, the origins of these exercises are shrouded in myth and legend. Some say the exercises began several thousand years ago. There are historical records of similar types of exercise dating back 4000 years to the time of the Yao settlements, when regulated body exercises and special breathing techniques were said to be used to cure disease. The most recent evidence of the long history of these movements comes from a silk book unearthed in 1979, known as the Dao Ying Xing Qi Fa (*Method of Inducing Free Flow of Chi*). The book dates from the Western Han dynasty, which ran from 206BC to AD24, and bears 44 drawings of men and women in exercise positions resembling those in this chapter.

Whatever the truth of the very ancient history of these exercises, it is known that the famous General Yeuh Fei who lived during the Southern Sung dynasty (AD1177-1279) developed a set of 12 fundamental exercises to train his army. These he later simplified to eight – Ba Duan Jin. The fact that he and his army were never defeated in battle was attributed to this training.

To this day, visitors to the famous Shaolin Temple in Henan, China, will see statues of monks performing Ba Duan Jin. The monks themselves use this system as part of their daily training.

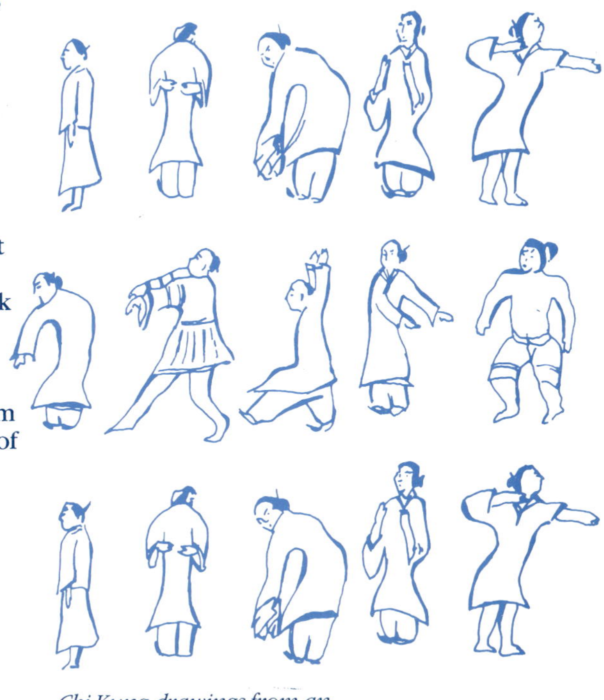

Chi Kung drawings from an original found in Dao Ying Xing Qi Fa.

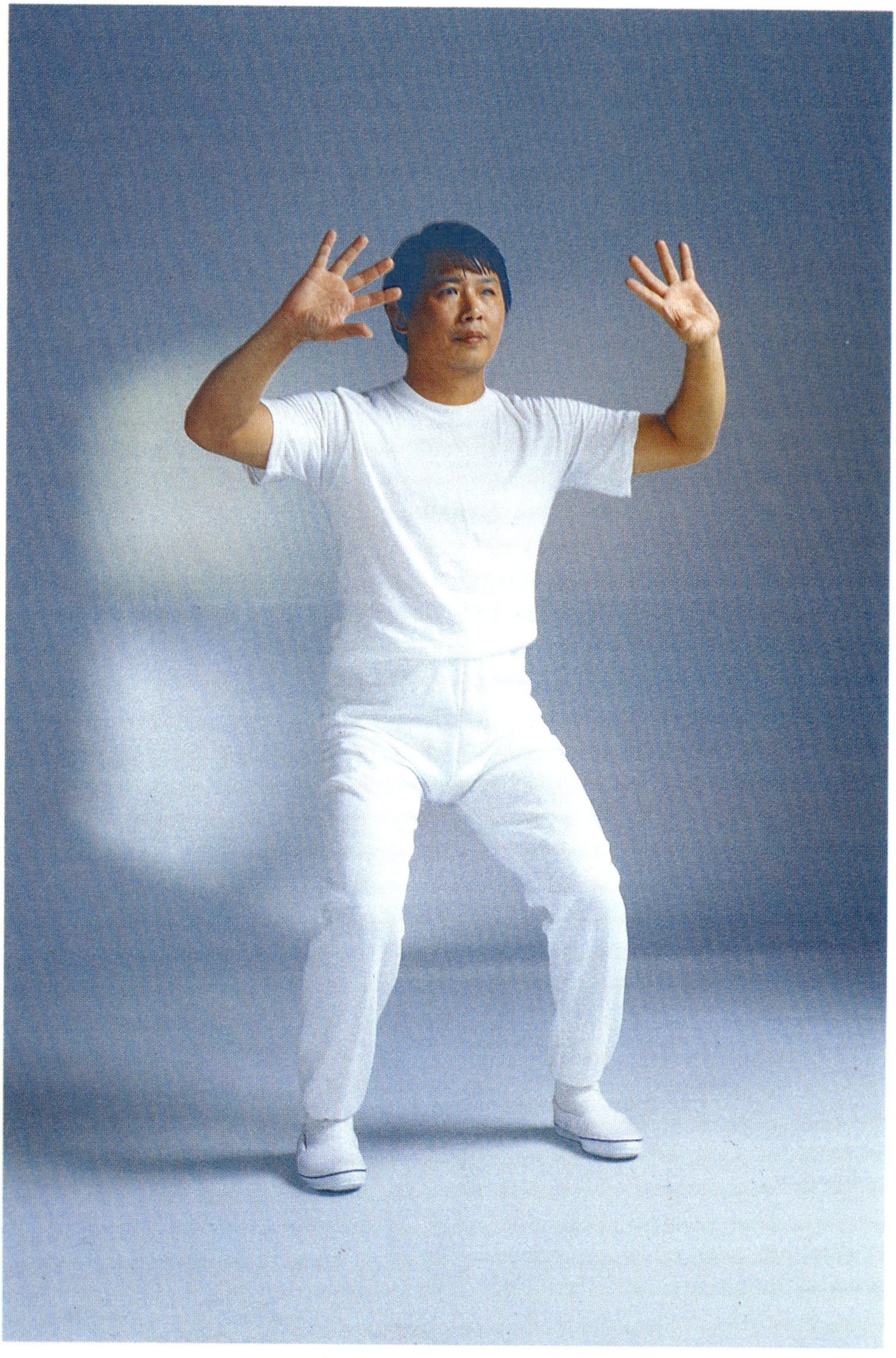

Master Lam in the fifth position.

CHAPTER 5
GROWING LIKE A TREE

Let us assume you have been practising Zhan Zhuang fairly regularly. Suppose it is six months since you first started. You find that you are able to stand in the second position – Holding the Balloon – for at least 20 minutes without having to lower your arms or stand up. The initial aching and trembling is gone. It is still not easy, but by relaxing and using the techniques for coping with your rebellious nervous system, you can sustain the posture. Now is the time to try the next three positions.

Start by doing the Ba Duan Jin exercises. You can add these to the very first warm up exercises for the knees and shoulders (see pp. 26-27) or go straight into them. Then stand for a few minutes in the first position – Wu Chi (see p. 29). Move gently into the second position – Holding the Balloon (see pp. 34-35) and stay there for 10 to 15 minutes. Then use the remaining time to start to learn the new positions outlined in this chapter.

First, add the third position – Holding your Belly (see pp. 84-85). Stay in the position for five minutes after the first exercises. After three weeks, reduce the time spent in the first and second positions and work up to 10 minutes in the third position. Aim toward holding it for up to 20 minutes after doing the Ba Duan Jin warm ups. Then do the same for the fourth position (see pp. 88-89), leaving out the third position for the time being.

The fifth position is extremely taxing (see pp. 92-93). Only a very highly experienced practitioner can sustain it for long periods. To start, just add a minute of it to the end of Holding the Balloon. Three weeks later, increase this to two minutes, and so on, aiming eventually for a period of five minutes.

Once you have completed the exercise in any of these positions, gently return to the original Wu Chi position. Stand quietly, allowing yourself to rest between heaven and earth.

As before, gently shake your arms and legs. Make a moderate series of arm circles and then finish with a little slow walking.

Holding your Belly – the third position

This position, in which your arms form a large, expansive downward curve, is a restful progression from Holding the Balloon. It is a powerful exercise in itself, and it also helps to gather the increased flow of Chi in your body and focus it on your Tan Tien (see p. 42).

The imaginary balloons that you held in the second position will also help you in this one. The balloons give you support and reduce the tension in your muscles (see also p. 98). By holding imaginary balls between your fingers you can create the same effect. An imaginary strap around your neck will lend additional support to your arms.

PREPARING FOR THE POSITION
Adopt the Wu Chi position (see p. 29), then bend your knees slightly as you would in the second position, lowering yourself about 5cm (2in). Keep your head, neck, torso, and pelvic girdle in the same relaxed, straight posture as in the first position.

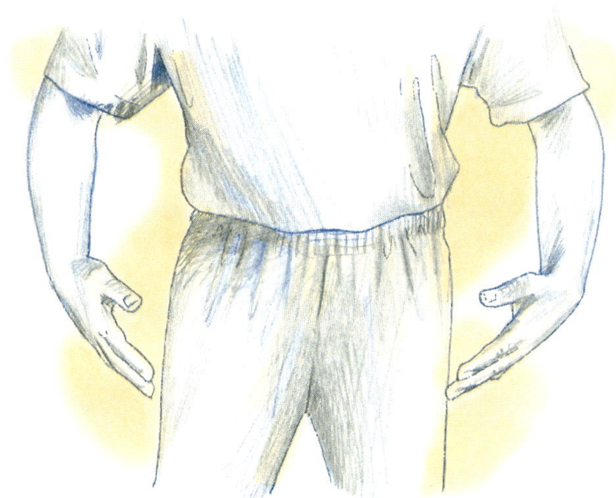

Slowly bring your forearms around in front of your abdomen. Raise and open your hands slightly and bring them to rest as if they were gently supporting an enormous belly that you had developed. Or you can imagine holding a large inflated balloon between your hands and your belly.

HOLDING YOUR BELLY

Your head remains suspended from the point in line with the tips of your ears (see p. 31). Your entire weight flows down from this point.

Your back remains straight, your knees bent. As you sink down about 5cm (2in), make sure your knees do not come forward beyond your toes.

Hold the imaginary balloon or your belly with your fingertips. The fingers of each hand point toward the opposite knee.

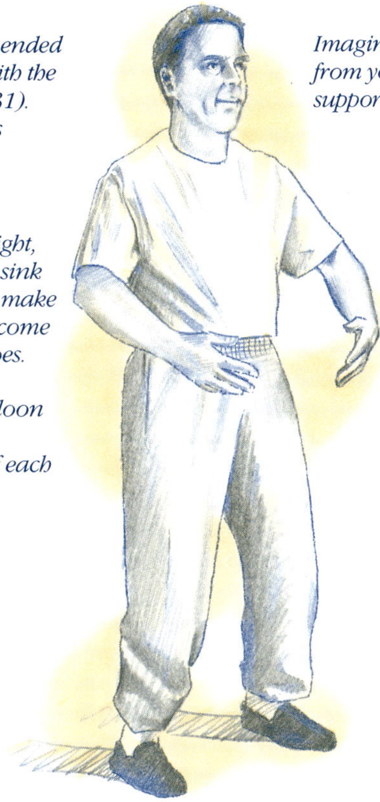

Imagine that a strap runs from your neck to your wrists, supporting them (see p. 99).

You hold your belly or a large balloon so gently that there is no tension in your wrists or fingers. Your palms are not turned sharply upward. They are loosely angled along the arc of the balloon or belly.

Keep your fingers separated just enough to allow little imaginary balls to rest between each of your fingers.

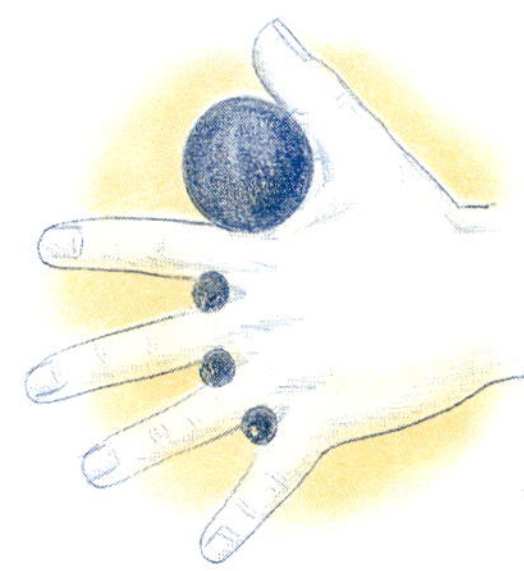

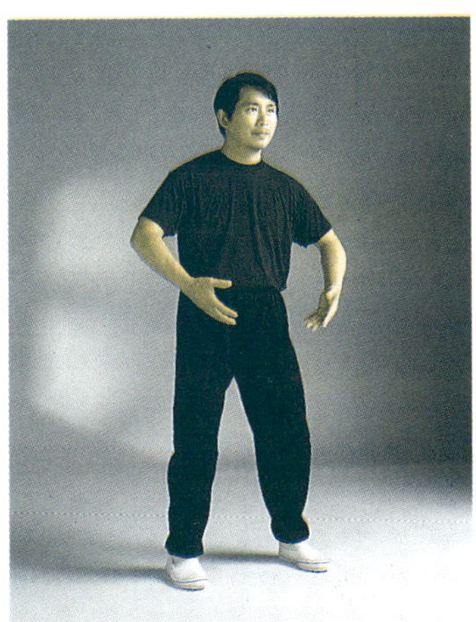

Master Lam in – the third position.

The Tree in the Harvest

The autumn sun is hot, the air is still. Long lines of sunlight filter through the orchards and across the golden fields. Small insects dart and hover in the warmth.

This is the time of bearing fruit. The tree has been transformed. It bore the patient work of summer's long, slow days. Now it is calm. Each leaf and living cell is rich.

The harvest has begun. The sound of labour drones across the land. The earth is yielding up its produce, like an offering.

Unmoved, the tree has stood in solitude, surrounded only by the universe. It did its work in silence. Now all its sinews store the essence it so soundlessly distilled from sunlight and from air.

Its spreading boughs are full, like woven baskets overfilled with fruit. The tree is heavy with its growth. The seeds of future forests lie in countless numbers in its arms.

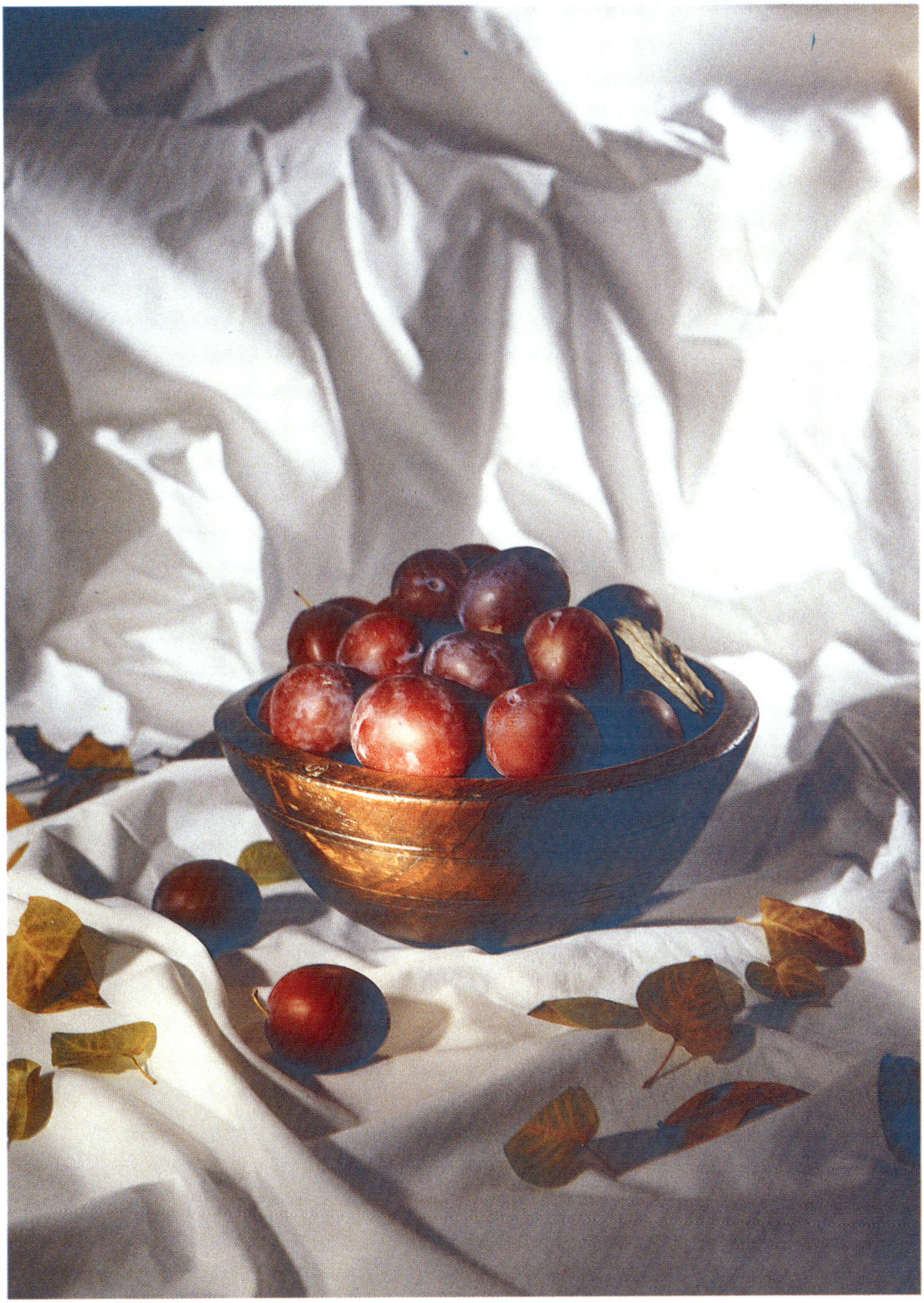

Standing in the Stream – the fourth position

Zhan Zhuang training advances in stages. Students progress from one position to the next at a careful pace. You should therefore move to this next position only when you feel you have become comfortable standing in the previous position for up to, say, 20 minutes. You are slowly building tremendous endurance. This next position will take you to a new level of stamina.

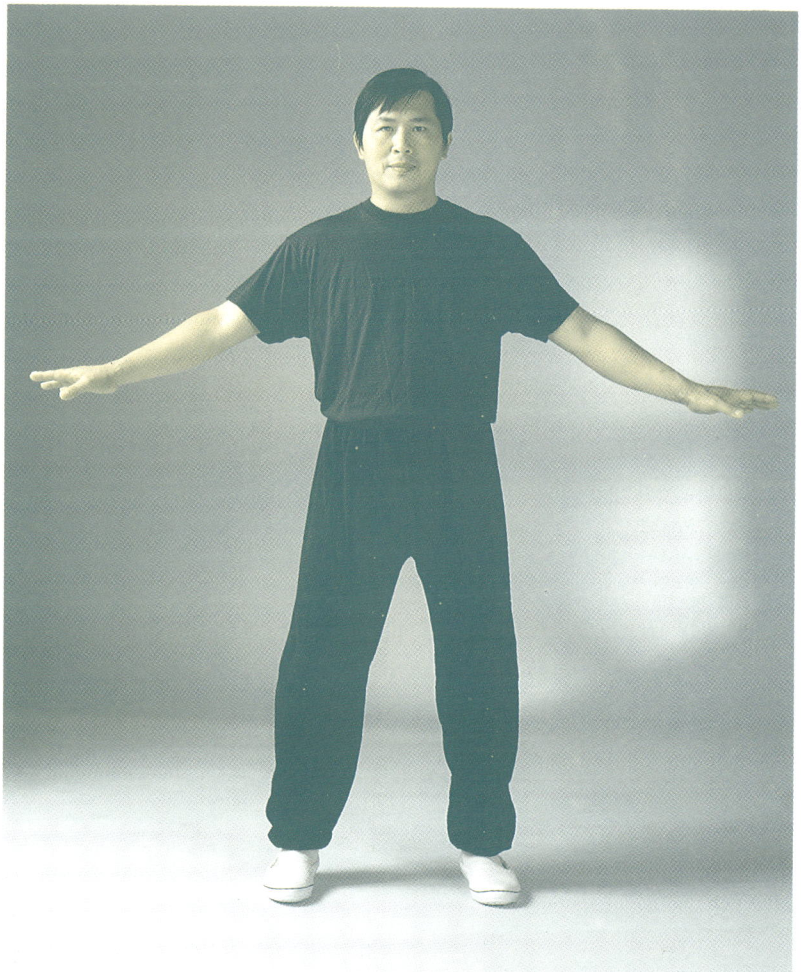

Master Lam in the fourth position

PREPARING FOR THE POSITION

Imagine that you are standing in a stream, with the current flowing toward you. Bend your knees, and sink down about 10cm (4in). Now reach your hands out to either side at waist height.

Imagine that you are suspended from the top of your skull, and that your wrists are supported by an invisible strap that runs from the back of your neck (see p. 99).

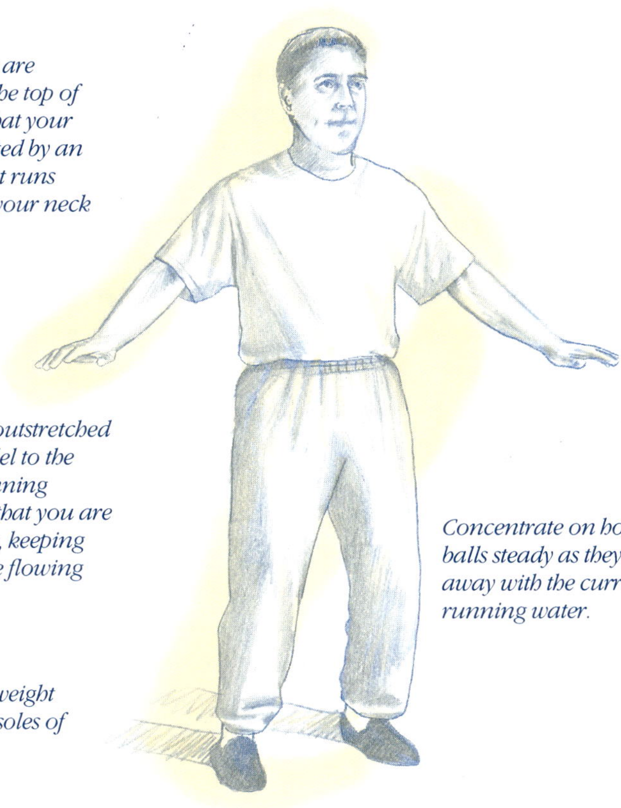

Your palms and outstretched fingers rest parallel to the surface of the running stream. Imagine that you are holding two balls, keeping them steady in the flowing water (see p. 99).

Concentrate on holding the balls steady as they try to float away with the current of the running water.

Imagine that all your weight is sinking down to the soles of your feet.

STANDING IN THE STREAM

The Tree in the Stream

The summer rain has washed the landscape. All the colours of the countryside are deeper than before. Dark, silent bushes glisten in the fields; the soil is black and wet.

The tree rises by the winding stream. It stands with arms outstretched as if at rest, while all that moves around it is in motion, like the mist.

The little stream is swelling in the flood. The rising currents in its depths are strong; the circles spinning on its surface are the work of countless raindrops.

The tree gives shelter to the rising stream. It stands alone as if it were a creature lost in thought. Its swaying boughs are balancing between the currents of the moving water and the wind.

The storm that drenched its bark is slowly passing and the distant sunlight slants between the clouds. The atmosphere is charged with countless particles. The tree is waiting, silently.

Just as the broad-winged falcon floats far above the valley, motionless, the tree is resting in the air. Its leafy branches hover in the light like flying creatures rising from the stream.

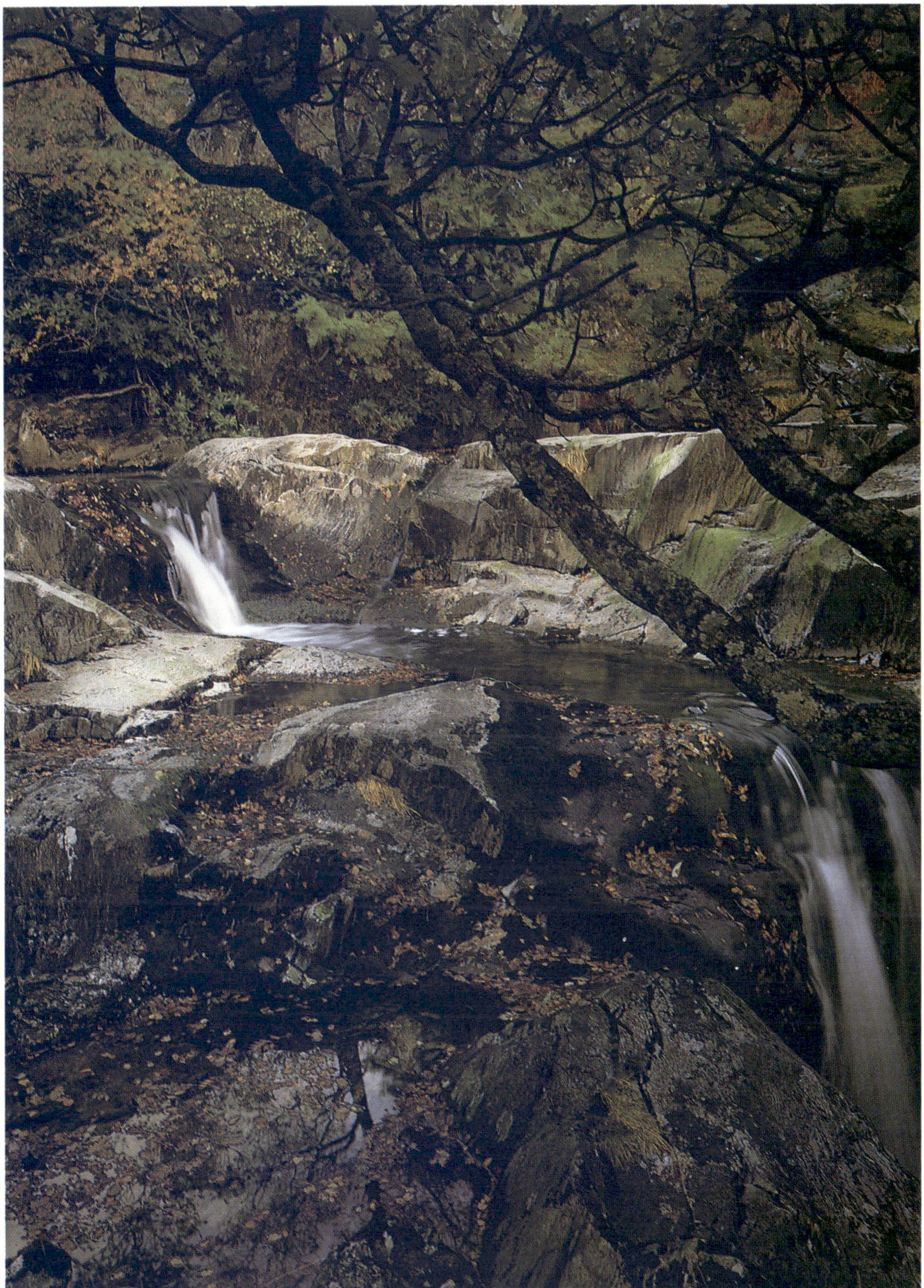

Holding the Balloon in Front of your Face – the fifth position

This next position is the most taxing so far. It places much greater demands on your legs and arms, and therefore requires a higher level of endurance.

Even after you have practised holding the first four Zhan Zhuang positions for some time, gradually increasing the duration as described, you will probably find this position extremely difficult to sustain. Many of your muscles will be almost certain to tense up and you may feel as if some are about to explode. You may well sweat profusely and begin to tremble (see Chapter 3). Don't use these initial sensations as an excuse for giving up. Use your mind to tell your muscles to relax and extend your endurance beyond the point of initial muscle exhaustion. Use the imaginary balloons to reduce tension and imagine, as before, that a strap around your neck is helping you hold your wrists in position (see p. 99).

PREPARING FOR THE POSITION
Sink down as deeply as you can manage – 20cm (8in) or more – being careful not to extend your knees over your toes. Bend as if you were sitting down, rather than moving forward to kneel. Your weight shifts a little toward your heels. You will immediately feel the pull on the muscles on the front of your thighs. Breathe normally.

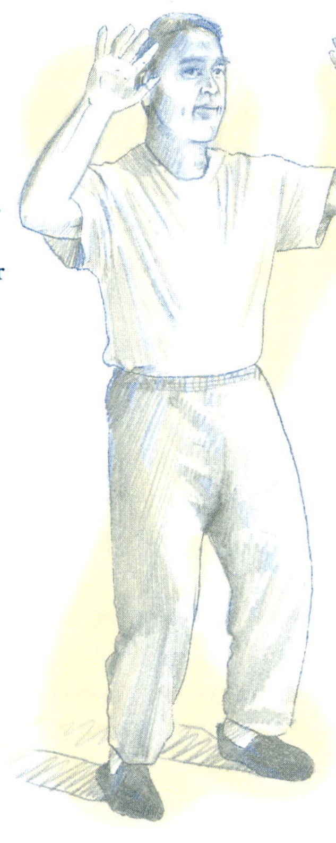

Raise your arms and turn your hands outward so that the backs of your hands are level with your cheeks.

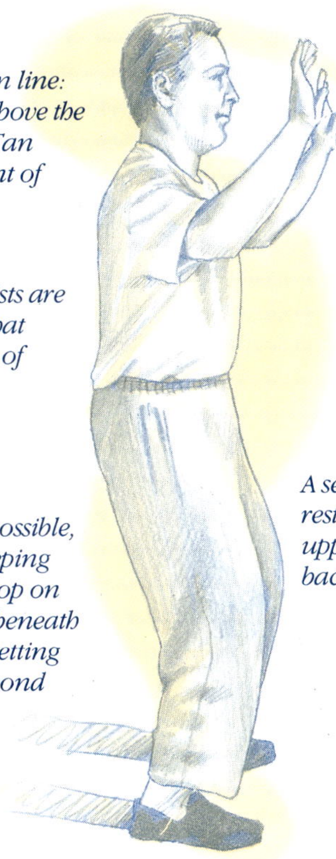

HOLDING THE BALLOON IN FRONT OF YOUR FACE

INCREASED ENERGY

The fifth position greatly increases the flow of energy in your body. You become like a bow in the moment before it releases the arrow, or like an athlete on the starting blocks waiting for the crack of the starting pistol. The effect is the result of pressure on your Chi circulation generated by the muscles in your legs – an effect you can feel while holding the posture and after you rise up to come out of it.

This is an extraordinarily demanding position to hold. Try not to bend forward at the waist too much. Do your best to relax your upper back and hips. That won't be easy at first, but over time you will acquire the physical and mental power to succeed.

The Tree in the Wind

Dark birds burst into flight. They dive and scatter in the wind.
High distant clouds trail long pale shadows on the earth –
the daylight changes with the moving sky.

The tree stands open to the heavens, touched by every
movement of the air. The driving wind curls round its leaves.
Its branches shake against the sky.

Gusts trace their flying patterns in the grass. The woody stems
of saplings sway and twist. Small bushes wave like slender
wands in children's hands.

The tree stands guard, its mighty limbs outstretched toward
the wind. Its roots are firm within the earth, its trunk is calm. It
is a place of shelter and it stands its ground.

Look! The silent tree has gathered up the current of the wind.
It floats in place like driftwood on the waves.

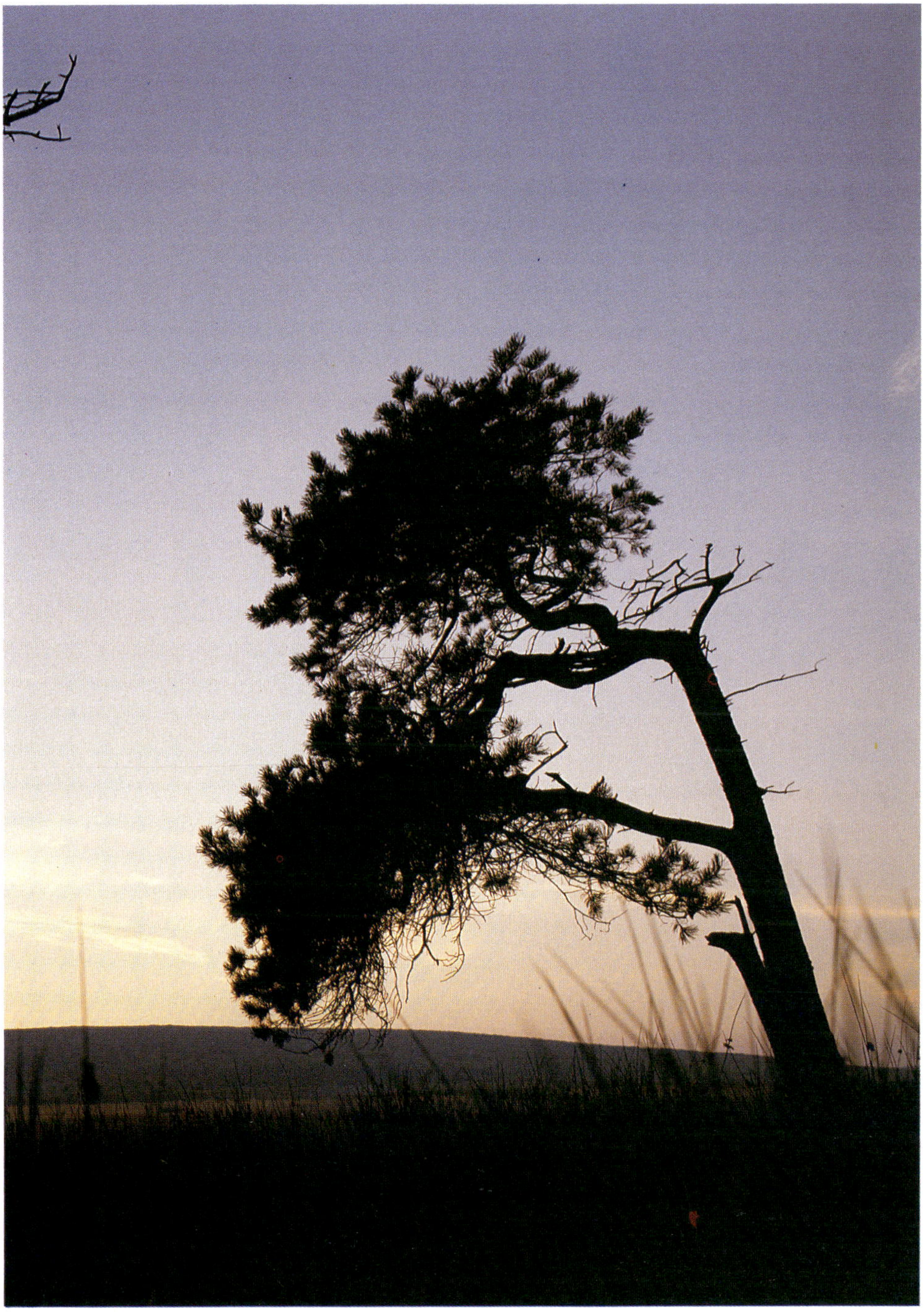

The Full Circle

This advanced exercise draws on all the basic Zhan Zhuang positions. Note that the sequence of movements is not in the same order as the sequence you have learned. It is based on the order that generates the maximum flow of energy. It should ideally be commenced only on the advice of your instructor.

You may find it a great help to put on some soft music for the duration of this exercise. If you put on a 30-minute tape, with a little practice you will be able to progress smoothly through the circle of positions in the correct time.

PRACTICAL TIPS

There are two other points to bear in mind: first, you can do the full circle with your eyes closed. Your closed eyes and the soft music will greatly aid relaxation through this intense exercise. Second, note that as you drop down in the second and fifth positions, your arms are in fact rising into higher positions, and that as you begin to rise up into the fourth and third positions, returning to the first position, your arms move into lower positions.

Begin in the first position – the Wu Chi (see p. 29). Then move gradually through the other four positions in the sequence shown on the facing page.

When you begin this exercise, hold the first position for two minutes, then the second position for five minutes, and then allow two minutes for each of the other positions, finishing with two minutes in the first position.

After you have reached this standard, move on to spend five minutes in each of the positions, finishing in the first position. This will take half an hour altogether.

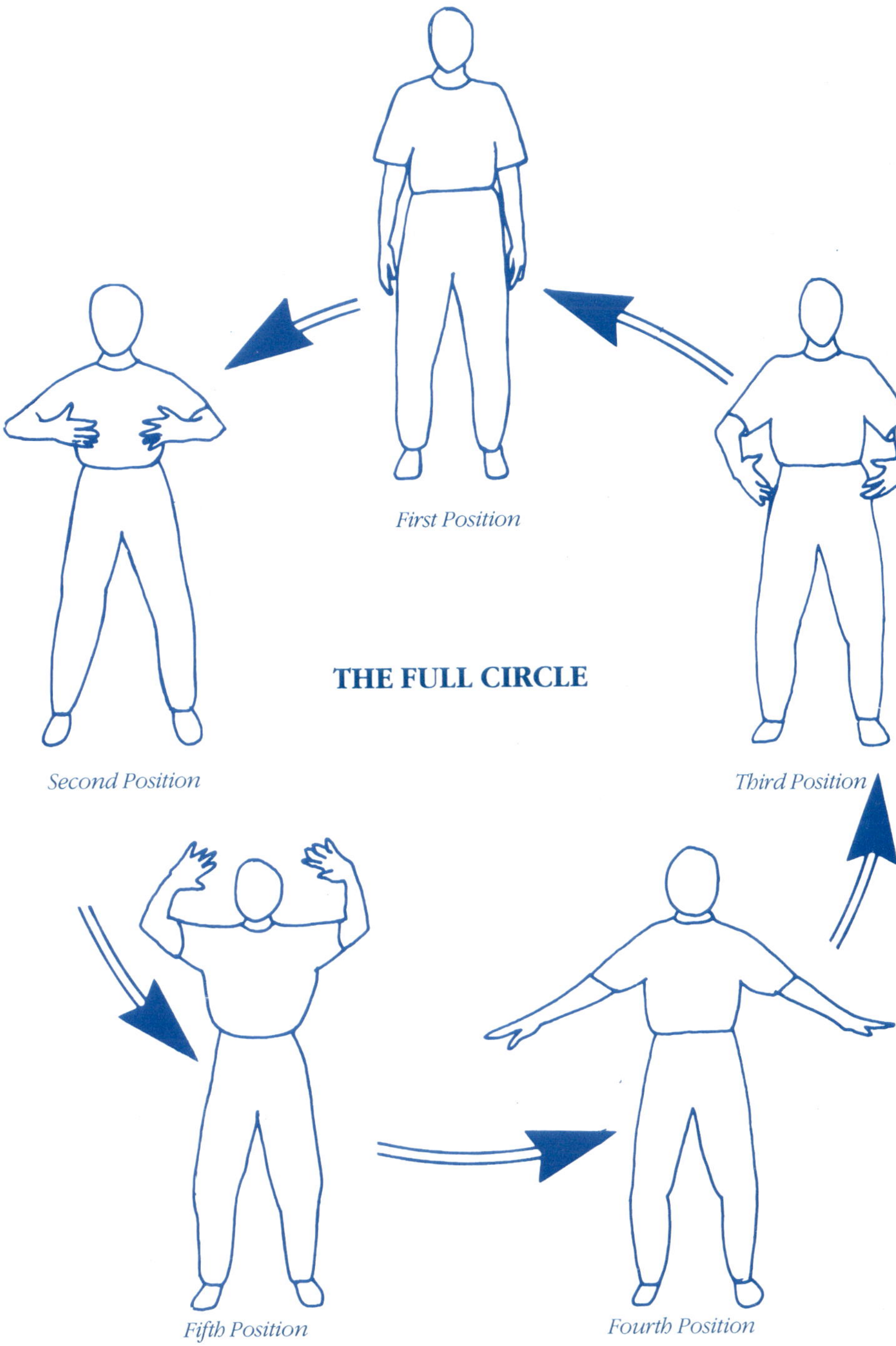
First Position
Second Position
THE FULL CIRCLE
Third Position
Fifth Position
Fourth Position

Understanding Zhan Zhuang

Students of Zhan Zhuang usually want to know all about the theory behind the practice, and where it will take them. "Are these exercises of any use?" "Am I hurting myself?" In the Orient, students must place their complete trust in their master. They know better than to question their teacher's unusual methods. In the West, this tradition of learning is largely unknown.

It may therefore help to give just a simplified explanation of what happens as you stand in these positions. As explained in Chapter 2, the Tan Tien is the focus of the Chi network in your body. It also functions like a reservoir. When you practise Tan Tien breathing, the Chi that you breathe in descends to this area. When the reservoir is full it acts like a pump, sending more and more Chi into a circuit around your body. It flows from the Tan Tien down your legs to your feet, then back up through your body to your arms, along your arms to your hands, and then back along your arms and neck up to your head. From there the circuit returns to the powerhouse of the Tan Tien.

The Zhan Zhuang positions enhance this flow. Raising and extending your arms reduces constraints on your internal organs and induces the Chi to flow into your hands and then up to your head. Bending your legs greatly increases the pressure of the Chi returning from your feet. All the Zhan Zhuang positions in this book, and the use of imaginary balloons and straps for support, are carefully designed to develop and adjust the flow of Chi along this circuit.

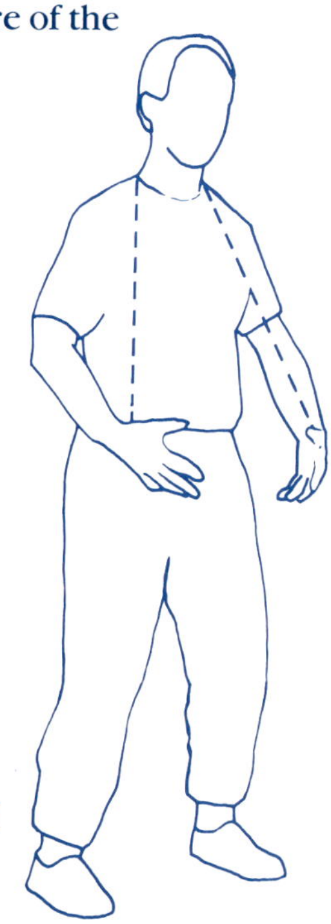

Imagine that a strap runs from your neck to your wrists, supporting them, and encouraging the flow of Chi.

Hold your belly, or a large, imaginary balloon, with your fingertips, so gently that there is no tension in your wrists or fingers.

THIRD POSITION

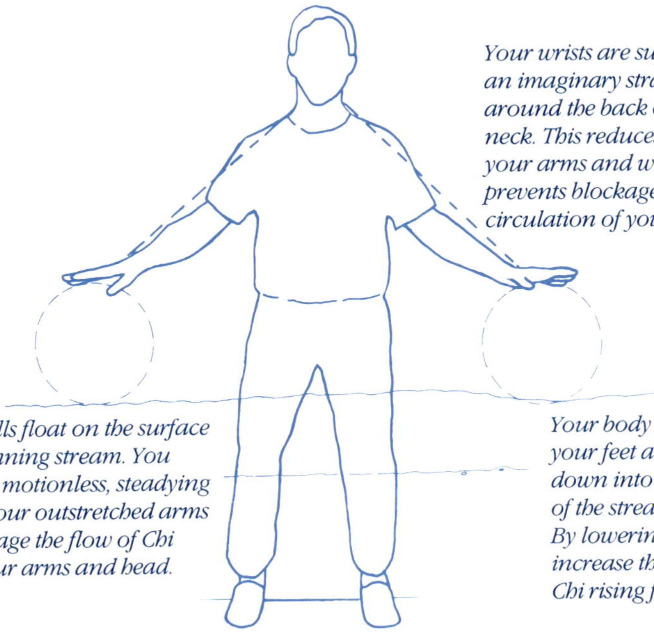

Your wrists are supported by an imaginary strap running around the back of your neck. This reduces tension in your arms and wrists, and so prevents blockages in the circulation of your Chi.

Two balls float on the surface of a running stream. You remain motionless, steadying them. Your outstretched arms encourage the flow of Chi into your arms and head.

Your body sinks down so that your feet and calves reach down into the soil of the bed of the stream and take root. By lowering your body, you increase the pressure of the Chi rising from your feet.

FOURTH POSITION

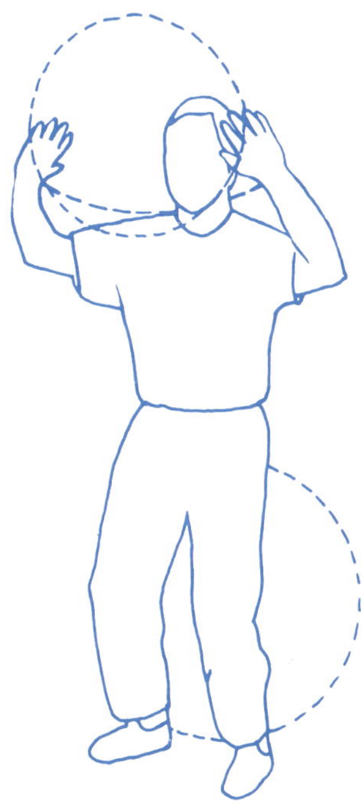

Imagine that your wrists are supported by a strap running around the back of your neck.

Imagine that you are pressing one balloon away from your face with your hands. This opens up the space under your arms, allowing the free flow of Chi.

Sink down as low as possible, dropping deeply into the balloon beneath your bottom for support.

FIFTH POSITION

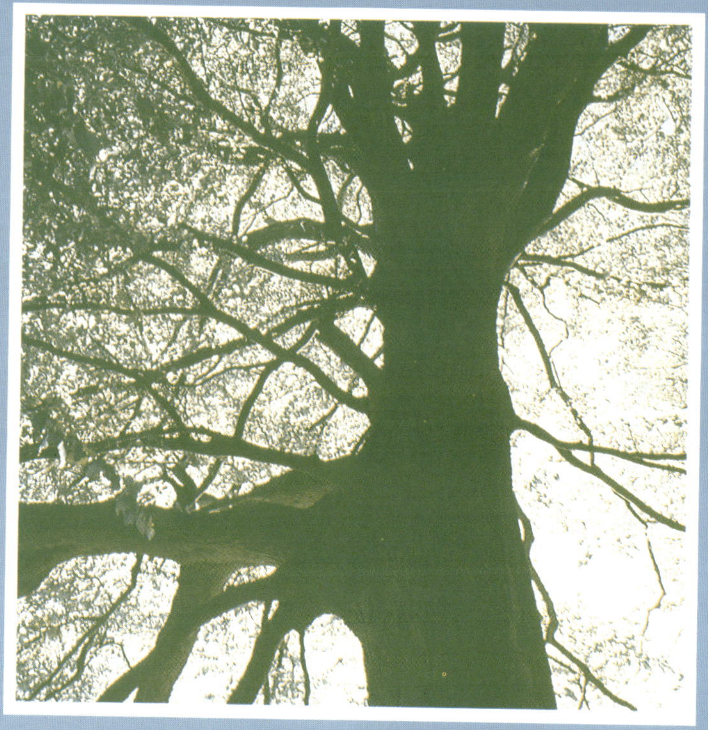

PART THREE

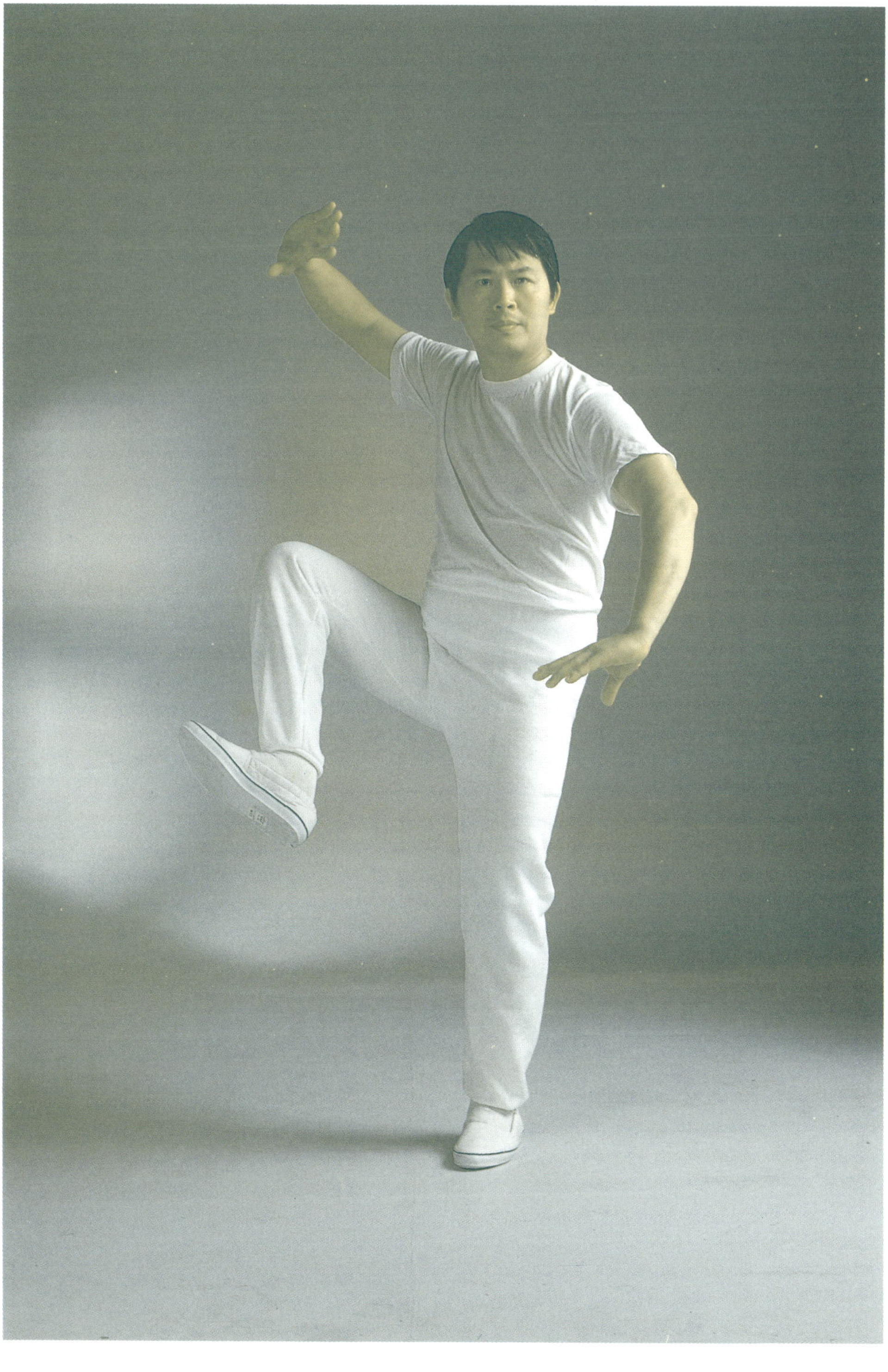

Master Lam in the ninth position.

CHAPTER 6
ROOTS AND BRANCHES

A tree experiences growth all over. New leaves grow every year. Twigs grow longer at their tips. Trunks and branches become thicker. The roots, too, thicken and lengthen. Zhan Zhuang training will also affect all parts of your body. This is partly because of the effect of the increased flow of Chi through the network of meridians, partly because of the strengthening of your cardiovascular and nervous systems, and partly because of the impact on various muscle groups. The Zhan Zhuang system helps you to extend the flow of your energy; it aims to fuse your whole being into a powerful, balanced force field.

The positions in this chapter help to extend the flow of Chi through your extremities. They are much harder to sustain for long periods than the exercises in Chapters 1 and 5. The exercises start to train you to be composed and stationary while standing with your weight shifted on to one side. The ninth position, at the end of the chapter, focuses your centre of gravity further to one side, with your weight rooted on a single foot.

Do not attempt the exercises in this chapter until you have become fully proficient at maintaining the positions outlined in Chapters 1 and 5. You are advised to attempt them only under the supervision of a qualified instructor.

Initially, you may have difficulty keeping still in any of these positions even for a minute or two. That is natural. Hold each position for as long as you can each time and slowly build up to longer periods as your body adjusts to the strain. Remember that you are growing from within – and that takes time!

The best way to add these new positions to your Zhan Zhuang training is to include them at the end of your basic standing exercise. For example, stand for 20 minutes in the second position – Holding the Balloon and then add two minutes of any of the positions outlined in this chapter. Then build from there.

Weight on One Leg – the sixth position

This position builds on what you have already learned. Having developed the ability to hold the first five positions, where the variation is chiefly in the position of your arms, you will now progress to shifting the alignment of your lower body. This position, as you will see, is an adaptation of the second to fifth positions. In each case, you shift your weight first on to your left leg, then your right. This means that you move through eight positions in all. Shift your weight in each position, first to the left and then to the right. Always stand for the same time on the left and right sides.

1. Begin by standing in the Wu Chi position (see p. 29). Relax thoroughly. Then bend your legs slightly, lowering yourself by no more than 5cm (2in). Arc your arms up to the second position – Holding the Balloon (see pp. 34-35). Let your upper body become weightless.

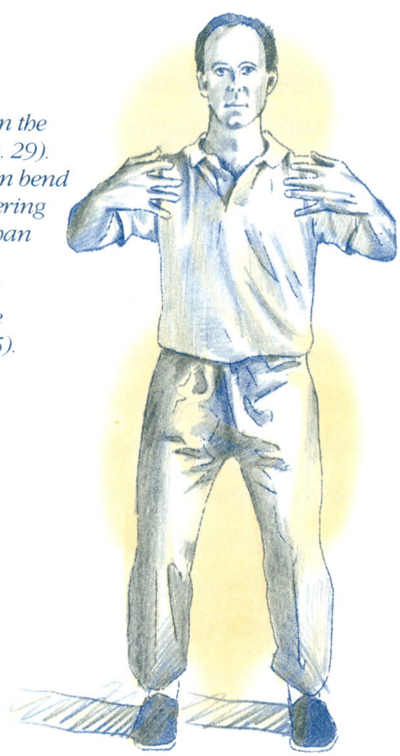

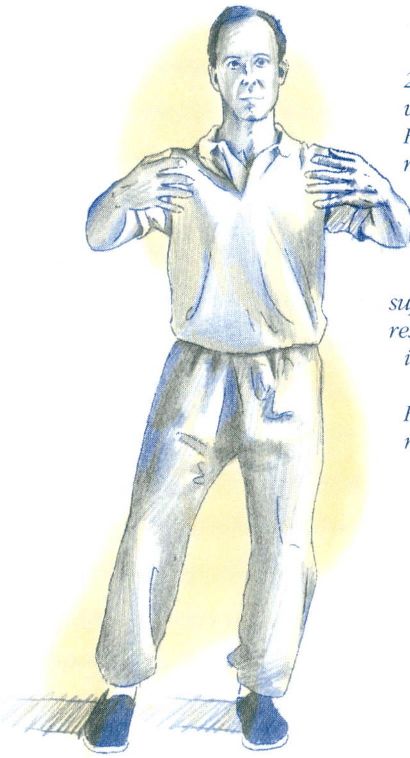

2. Now slowly shift your entire weight on to your left leg. Forget completely about your right leg. It is simply there, as it was before, but your mind and weight are entirely in your left leg. Imagine that your left buttock is supported by a huge balloon resting beneath it and taking its weight.

Hold that position for a minute or two. Do not move.

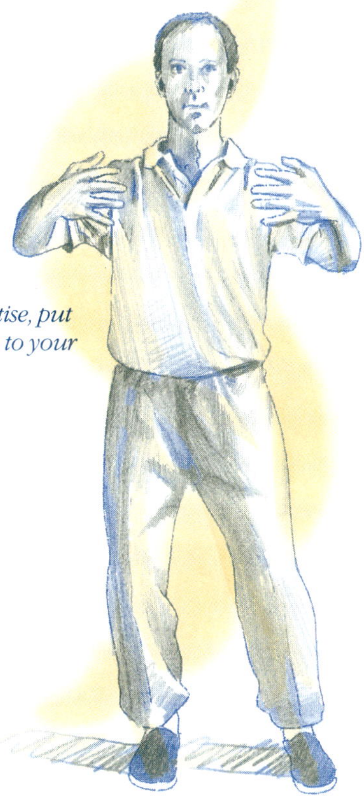

3. Next time you practise, put your entire weight on to your right leg.

The sixth position – variations

The next six variants on this position are achieved as you place your hands in each of the subsequent Zhan Zhuang positions: Holding your Belly (third position), Standing in the Stream (fourth position), and Holding the Balloon in Front of your Face (fifth position). Do each, first of all placing your full weight on your left leg and the next time on your right leg.

PRACTICAL TIPS

Do not sink lower than 5cm (2in) in any of these positions when placing your weight on one leg. Just concentrate on standing still and unwavering on the one leg and dispelling all tension from the rest of your body. Review the charts on pages 35 and 98 to 99 for each position, to ensure that all the details for the correct arrangement of your hands, arms, shoulders, neck, and head are fresh in your mind. Make sure that you observe all these points while holding the positions with your weight on one leg. The order in which you work through the positions is unimportant.

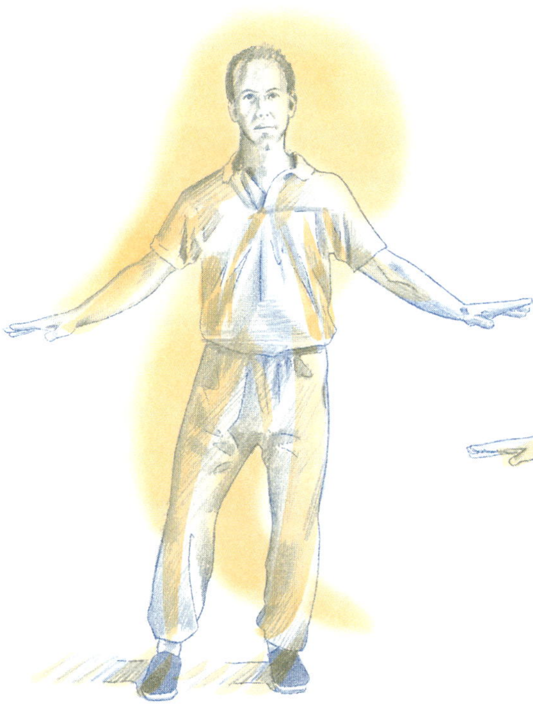

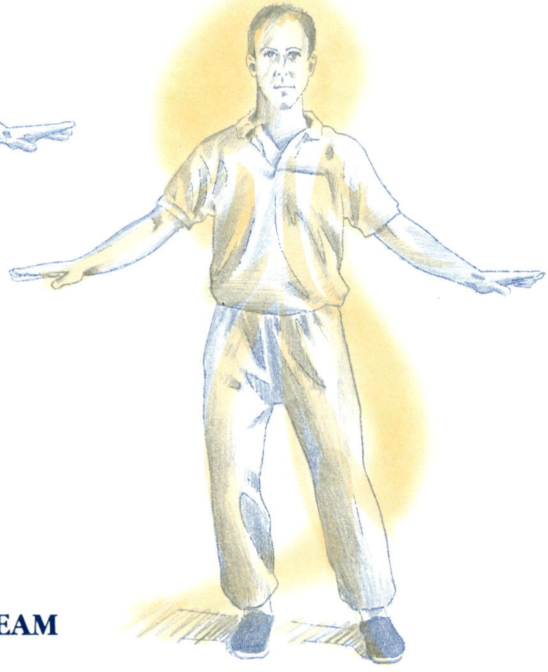

STANDING IN THE STREAM

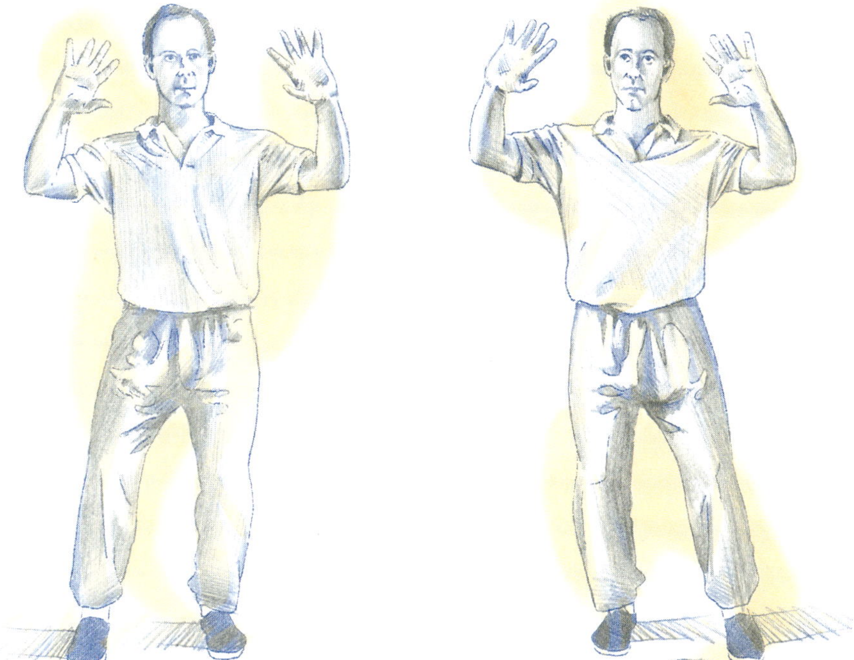

HOLDING THE BALLOON IN FRONT OF YOUR FACE

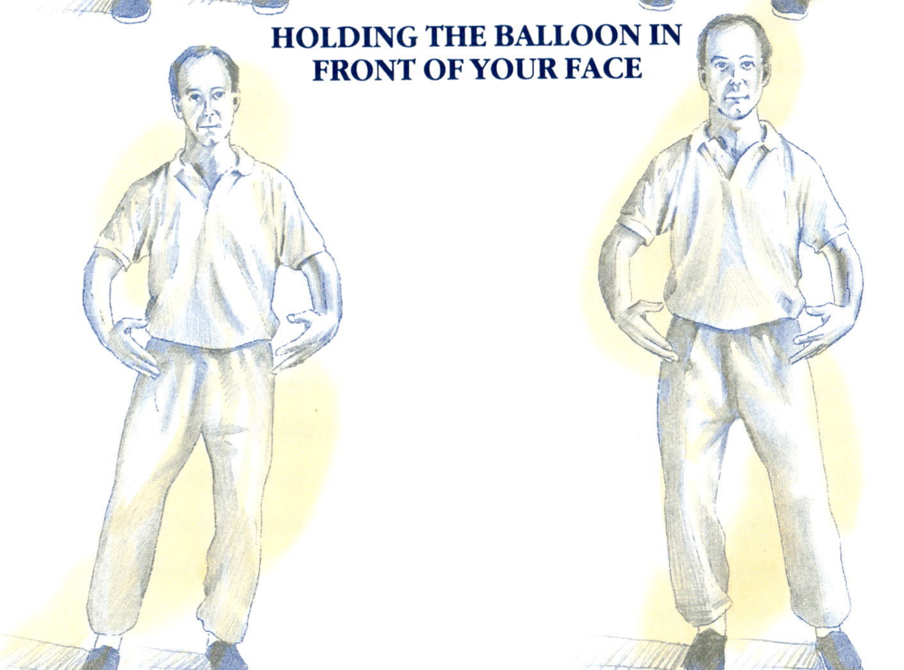

HOLDING YOUR BELLY

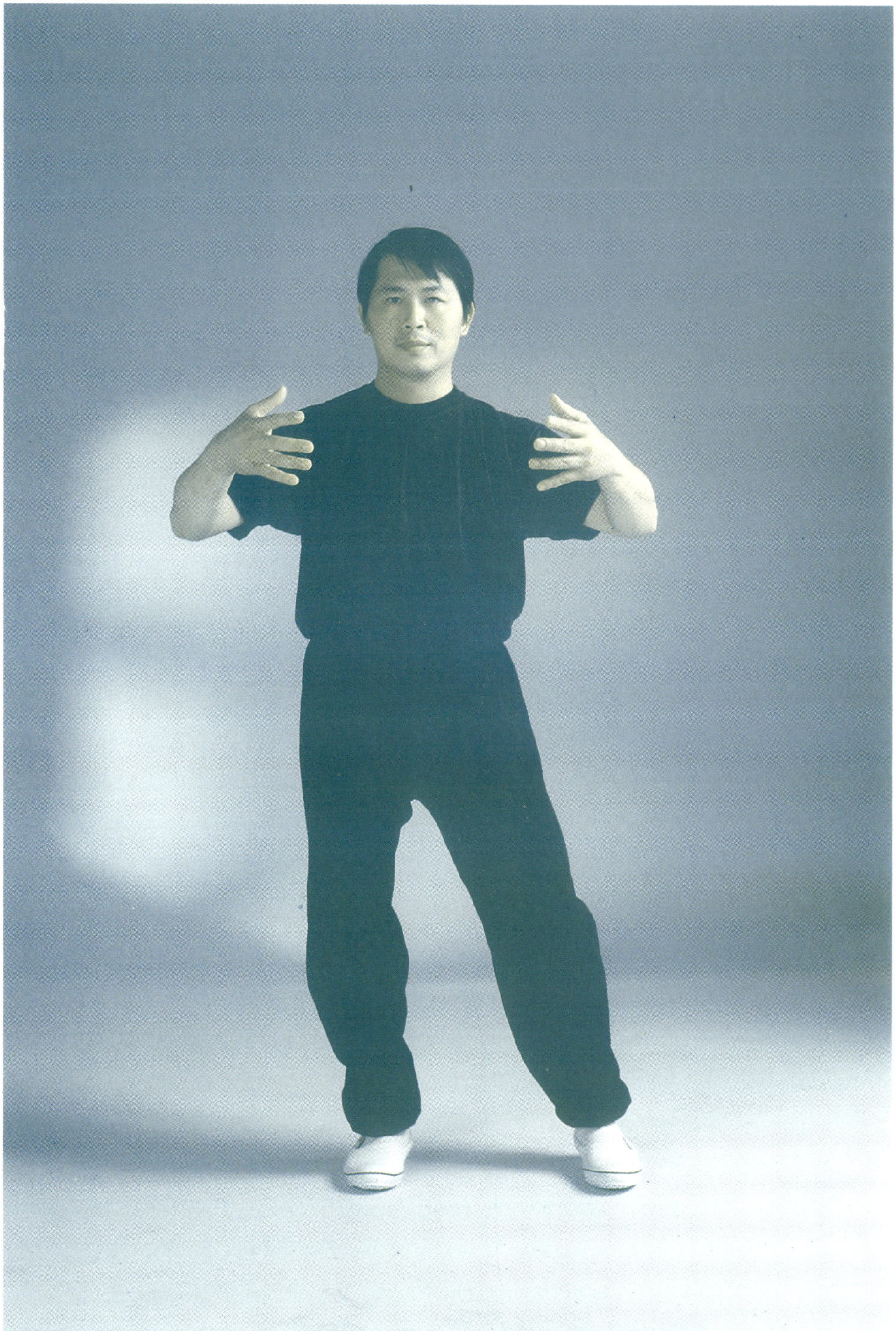

Master Lam in the sixth position.

Shifting your Weight

There are two variations on the initial two standing positions that will help strengthen the muscles of your legs. They involve shifting your weight forward and backward. By leaning slightly forward you strengthen your calf muscles. By leaning backward you develop the muscles in your thighs. Increasing the power of both muscle groups is important for your future progress in the Zhan Zhuang system.

A variant is to shift your weight from one side to the other so that you stand with 90 per cent of your weight on one leg.

1. Stand in any of the Zhan Zhuang positions you wish. The second position – Holding the Balloon – is most commonly chosen. Distribute your weight equally over both your feet.

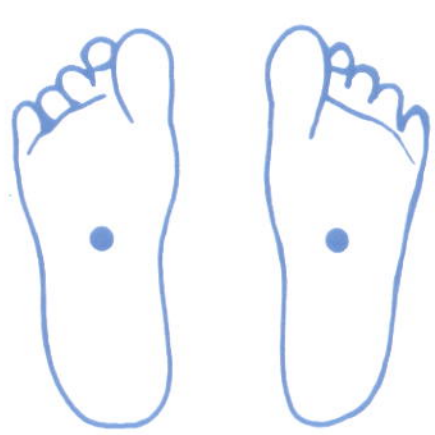

1. Weight over the middle of your feet.

2. As you stand, shift your weight forward on to the balls of your feet. Your heels should rise slightly, so that you could just slide a piece of paper under them. Stand with your full weight in that position.

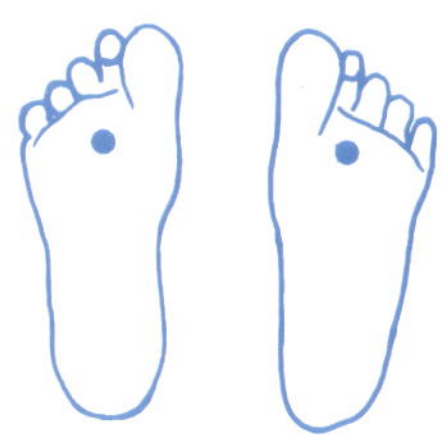

2. Weight on the balls of your feet.

3. After a minute or two, slowly rock backward. Let all your weight flow down into your heels. Lean backward almost to the point of losing your balance and use your toes to grip the floor or insoles of your shoes to keep you from falling. Now sit down on an imaginary beach ball behind you. Drop down as far as possible, as if sitting down in a chair. Keep your knees directly above the tips of your toes (see p. 93).

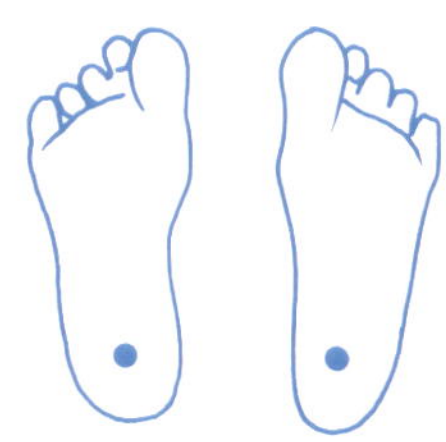

3. Weight on your heels.

The Bamboo Bears the Weight

The temple junipers have stood for many years and countless travellers have rested in their shade. Now they are ageing. Their ponderous boughs begin to droop and break.

Nearby, a mighty oak lies fallen in the woods: a century of growth uprooted in a sudden moment, like a twig.

Beyond the trees rise the tall bamboos. Like flying cranes, they stand at rest. One slender leg sustains them imperturbably between the grasses and the open sky.

In early spring the sun streams through their thin green leaves. Young shoots stretch up toward the brightness overhead. Their parents wave in sunlight far above.

The sound of wind comes from the woods. As if they were a thousand swaying hands, the leaves on all the shafts turn slowly in the air.

Beneath its sloping shoots, the bamboo's stem is gently curved. It takes the force of all the elements – enduring, rooted, calm. Unlike the trees that break and fall, its stem is just a hollow, nothing more. Its strength is in its emptiness.

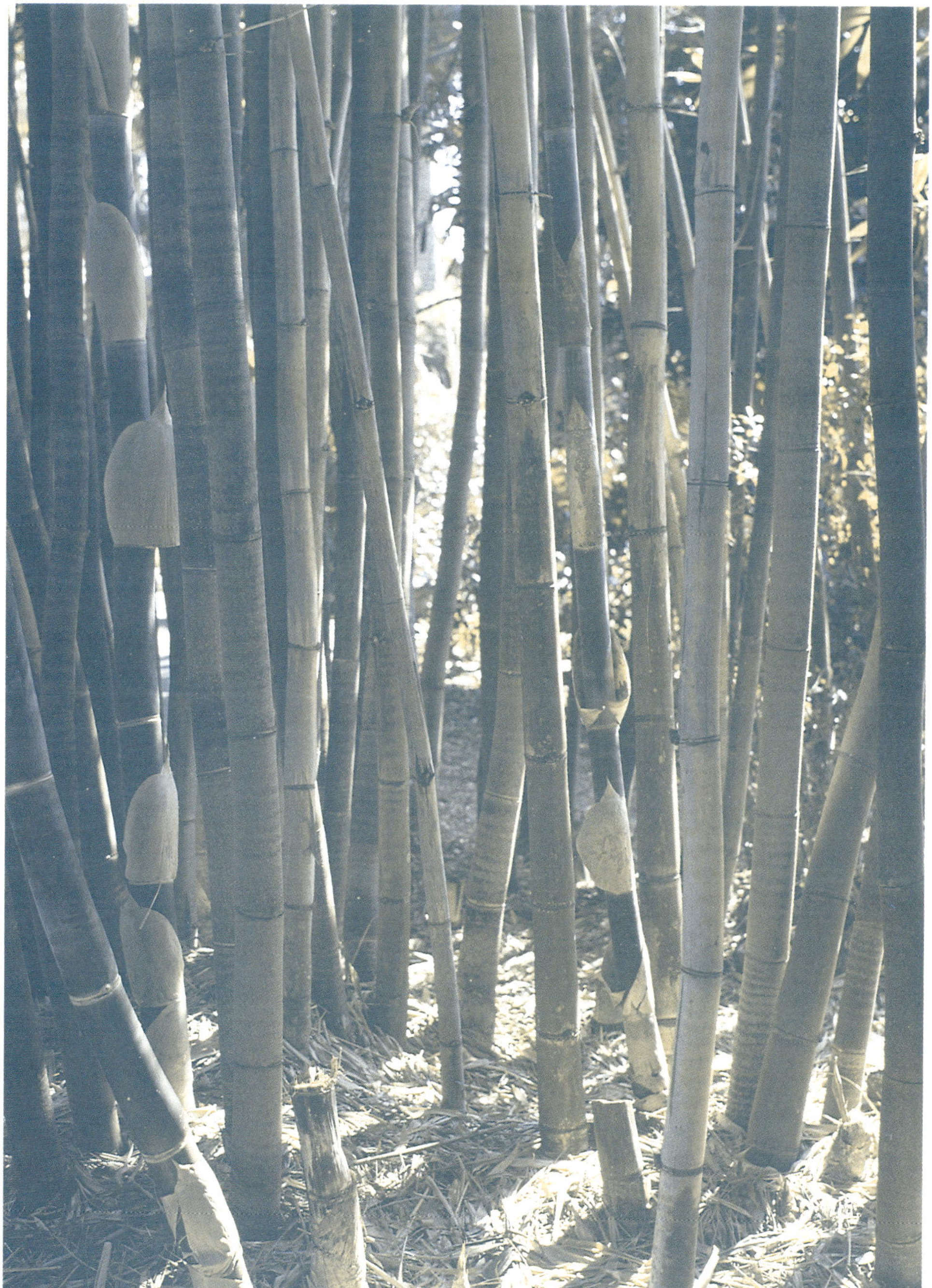

Holding the Ball on One Side – the seventh position

Begin by adding the seventh position to the end of standing in the second position – Holding the Balloon (see p. 35), and gradually increase the time you allocate to the new position to one or two minutes. At the end of the exercise turn back slowly to Holding the Balloon, then gently lower your arms and finish in the Wu Chi position (see p. 29).

Check that you are relaxed: rest comfortably on the imaginary balloons that support you.

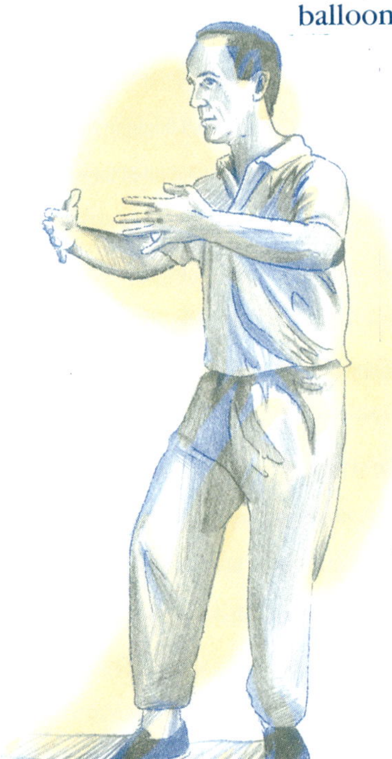

PREPARING FOR THE POSITION

Adopt the second position – Holding the Balloon (see p. 35). Make sure your neck and shoulders are relaxed and that there is space between your fingers to hold little imaginary balls between them. Imagine that there are balloons beneath your armpits and elbows, between your thighs, and under your bottom, gently supporting your weight.

1. Now turn your hips and torso slowly to the right. Allow your right heel to rise slightly off the ground (as if making space for a pencil) but keep your right toes lightly in contact with the ground: they turn with you as you move. Your weight will start to shift naturally on to your left leg. Turn through 45 degrees to the right. Let your head and eyes turn with your torso.

Hold that position, all weight fully on your left leg, for one or two minutes without moving (see left).

2. You should also practise this position on the opposite side, with your weight fully on your right leg (see right).

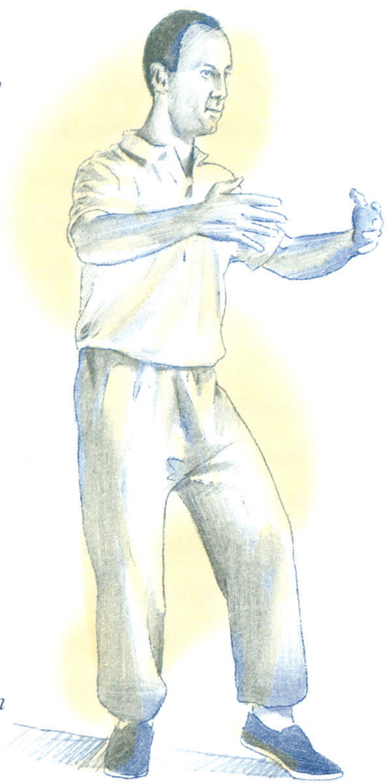

The Tree Grows to the Side

It is late autumn in the mountains. The broad-leaved trees are bare. Pale mosses grow beside the rocks. On distant peaks, the winds are raising plumes of snow.

Among the weathered rocks a solitary pine is standing in the wind. Its back is to the mountain side. Its branches turn toward the valley, like arms around the streams of rising air.

The pine knows that the frost is coming as the frost has come before. Where tiny pine flowers bloomed in spring, now cones have formed around the seeds.

It will take years before the pine seeds ripen. There is nothing to be done. The tree is growing like a forest. It gazes outward from the mountain side, a parent waiting for a birth.

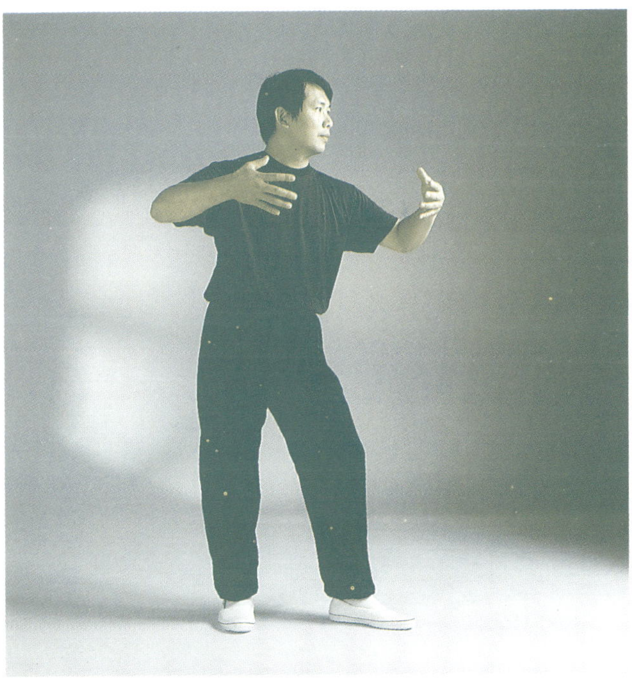

Master Lam in the seventh position.

Extending One Foot Forward – the eighth position

In this position, the pressure on the leg bearing most of your weight is greatly increased. It takes a long time to build up the strength, balance, and stamina required to sustain the posture. Don't try to get around the physical and mental obstacles – just persist, constantly being alert to your position and telling your muscles to relax.

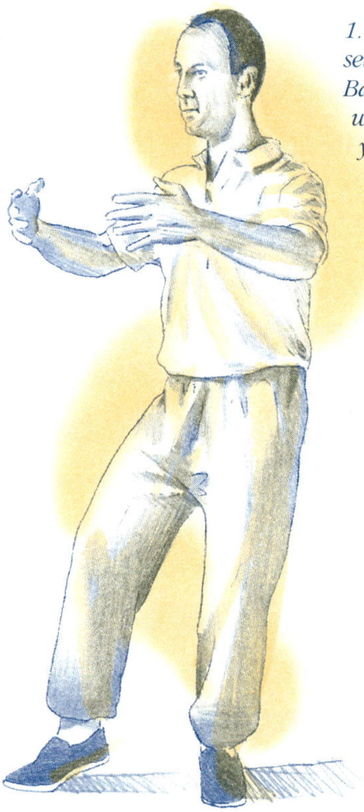

1. To begin, stand in the seventh position – Holding the Ball on One Side (see p. 112), with your weight fully on your left leg. Bend your left knee slightly to lower yourself by a further 5cm (2in).

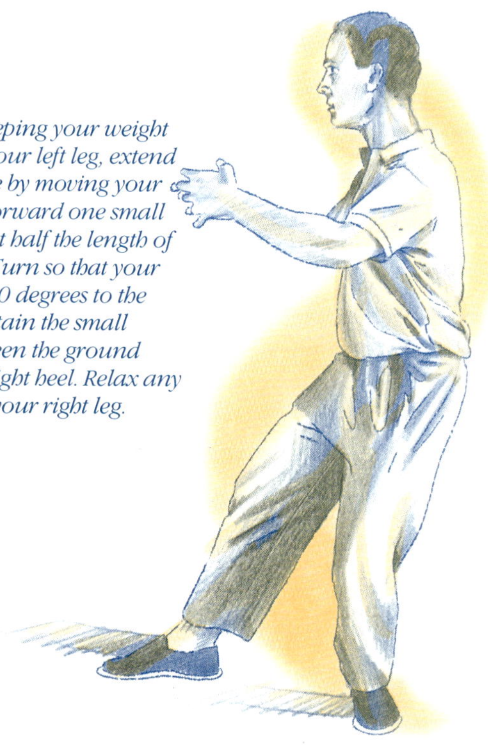

2. Then, keeping your weight rooted in your left leg, extend your stance by moving your right foot forward one small step – about half the length of your foot. Turn so that your foot faces 90 degrees to the right. Maintain the small space between the ground and your right heel. Relax any tension in your right leg.

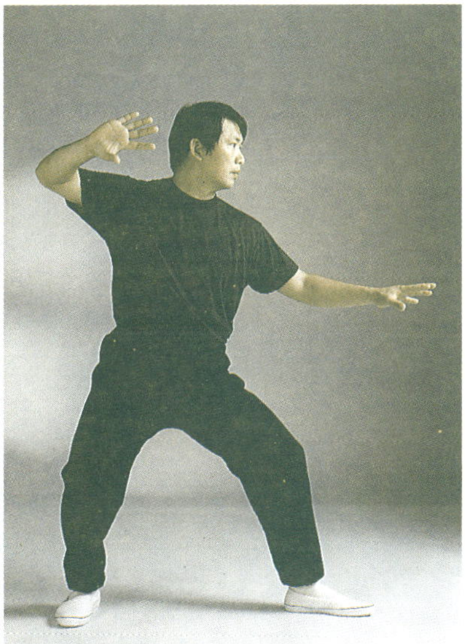

Master Lam in the eighth position

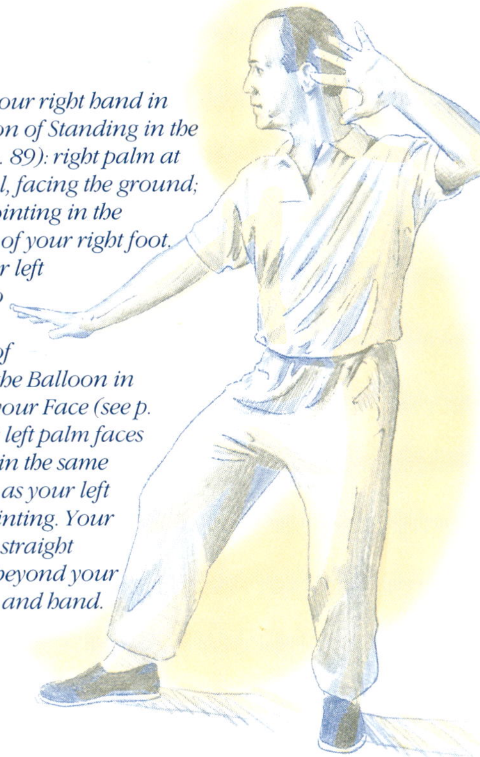

3. Place your right hand in the position of Standing in the Stream (p. 89): right palm at waist level, facing the ground; fingers pointing in the direction of your right foot. Raise your left hand into the position of Holding the Balloon in Front of your Face (see p. 92). Your left palm faces outward in the same direction as your left foot is pointing. Your eyes look straight forward beyond your right foot and hand.

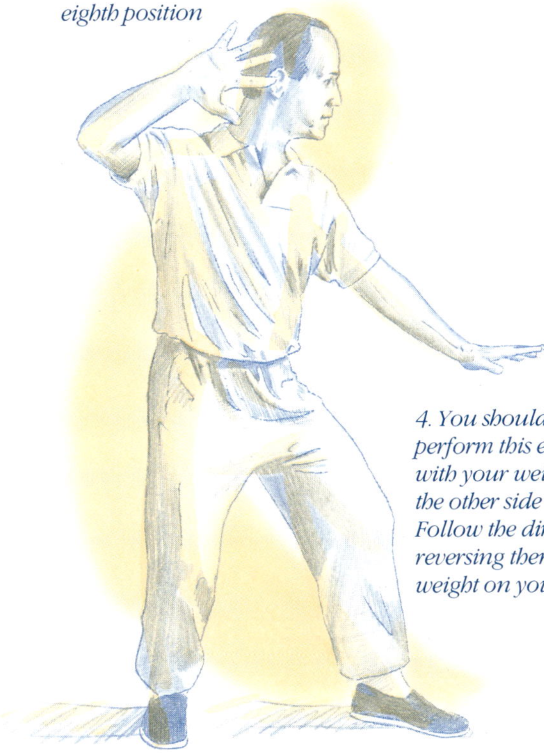

4. You should also perform this exercise with your weight on the other side (see left). Follow the directions above, reversing them to put your weight on your right leg.

The Tree Sends Out its Roots

The tree is growing in a courtyard. Early morning sunlight glances off the stones and porcelain tiles. The shrubs among the rocks are wet with dew.

Stone walls surround the courtyard on all sides. The tree and all that grows within the confines are unmoving, held like stately prisoners in their places. Small birds move out along the branches and are gone.

The silence and the stillness mask the tree's persistent work. It stands beside the stonework, motionless, but underneath the ground its roots are seeking out new soil.

The work is hidden, delicate. The tiny root hairs reach into the dark. The tender tip of every filament is inching outward in the earth.

Soon gardeners will come to tend the jasmine and the hyacinth. The day will bring the sounds of many visitors. Now, in the precious hours of the dawn, the little garden stands alone.

The spreading tree is breaking through the wall. Like little raindrops seeping through the rocks, its patient roots are boring through the stone. The layered mortar splits apart and cracks, while overhead a thousand leaves breathe, silent in the light.

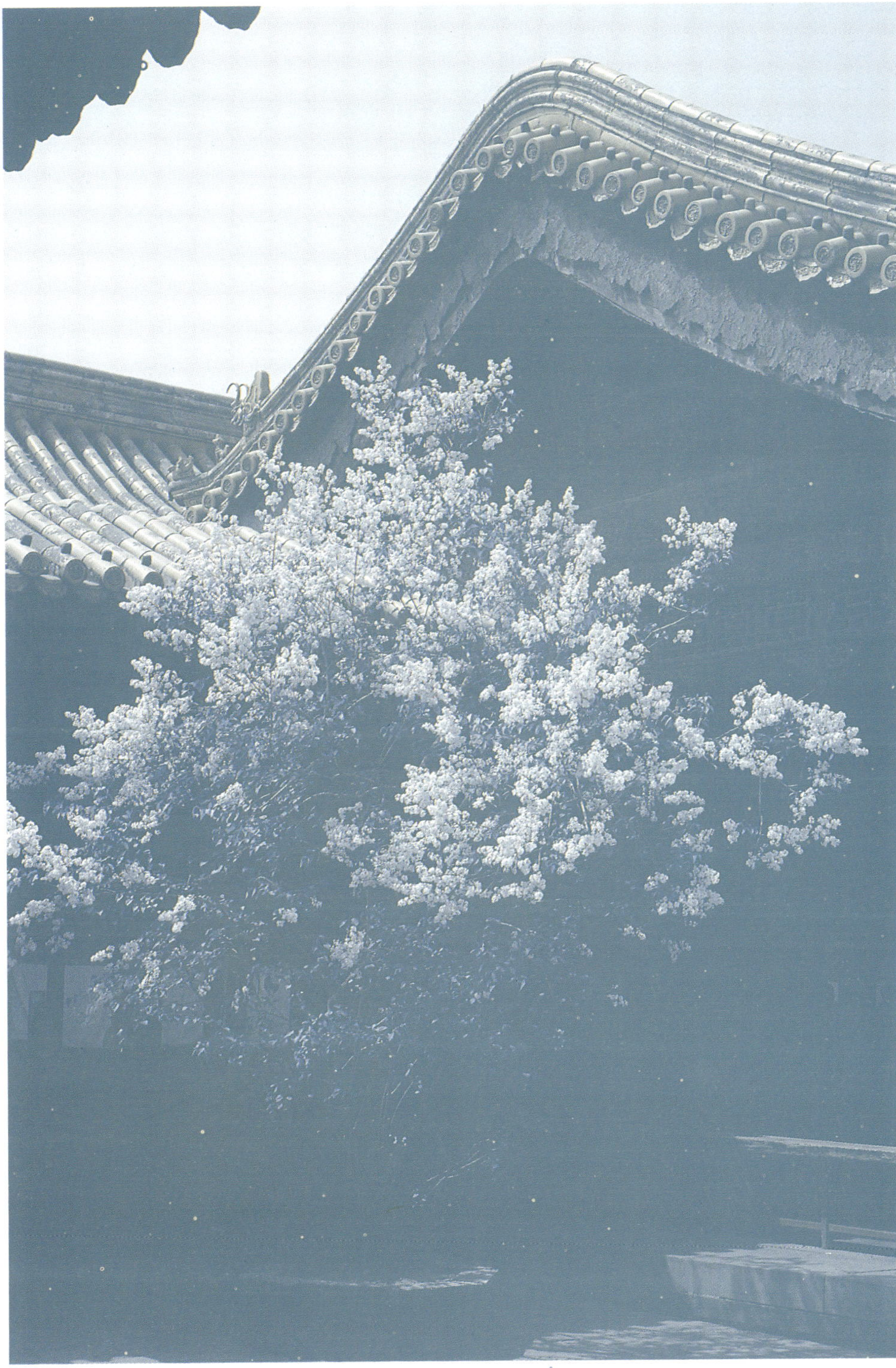

Rising Up on One Leg – the ninth position

This is the most advanced physical stage of the Zhan Zhuang training presented in this book. Do not attempt it until you are comfortable with the previous positions. There is no point in straining your muscles and exhausting yourself by trying out such advanced exercises without having carefully laid the internal foundations. There is an advanced stage to this last position (see facing page); this will greatly increase the benefits of the position to your energy system.

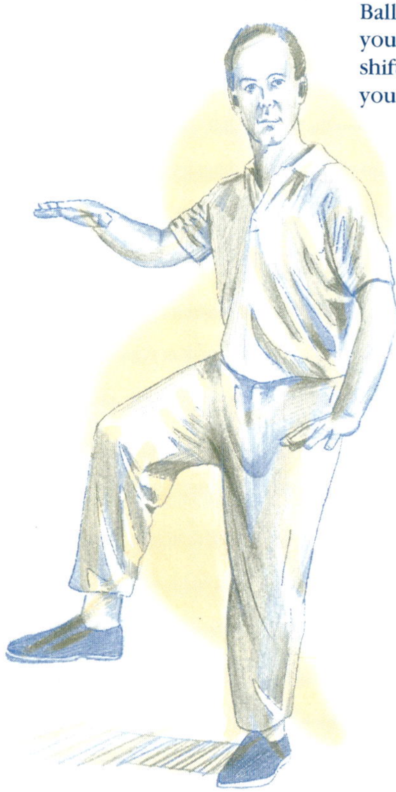

PREPARING FOR THE POSITION

Relax thoroughly before you begin. Assume the second position – Holding the Balloon (see p. 35). Lower yourself by 5cm (2in). Slowly shift your entire weight on to your left leg.

Raise your right arm and right leg together, as if an invisible string were stretched between them. Lift your right knee level with your waist, and your right palm level with your shoulder, facing downward. Your foot should be parallel to the floor. At the same time, lower your left hand to waist level, palm parallel to the ground.

Turn your head to the left so that your eyes are looking along the left diagonal. Complete the position by gripping the ground firmly with your toes.

REPEAT THE EXERCISE

Do this exercise to the other side as well, standing firmly on your right leg and raising your left arm and leg.

THE SECOND STAGE

When you can maintain this position without losing your balance, you can increase the benefit of the exercise by making the adjustment shown below.

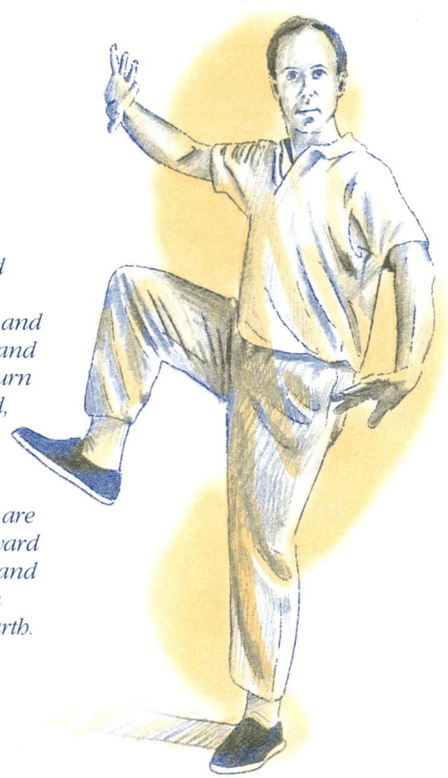

As you raise your foot and hand, stretch your toes upward as far as you can and turn your palm outward and upward toward the sky. Turn your lower hand outward, as if pulling away from your body.

Your raised arm and foot are being drawn upward, toward the heavens. Your lower hand and foot are being drawn downward, toward the earth.

RELAX AND REPEAT

You cannot stand in this advanced position for very long – probably less than half a minute to begin with, building up to a few minutes over many months of practice. Relax back to the first stage (see left), palms and foot parallel to the ground. Then expand again into the advanced position. Complete this cycle several times. Then rest in the third position – Holding your Belly (see p. 85) for one or two minutes.

The Tree Grows Out from the Cliff

The night is slowly giving way to day. The mist is lifting from the mountain side. The woods are silent, waiting for the dawn.

Above them is the rock face, rising overhead. High up the cliff, a mighty tree is growing on the stone. Its roots, like giant coils of rope, stretch out across the mountain ledge and down the veins of rock.

The day's first light begins to warm the morning air. The summer's heat will soon be full. All day the tree must bear the sun's full force, its branches arching outward in the sky.

Far below it stretch the woodlands and the mountain river beds. For miles, the hillsides rise in rows and then the valleys rich with villages and fields.

As if its boughs protected all the creatures of the hills, the tree stands like a sentinel, serene and fearless on the rock. The sun's first rays have reached its topmost boughs. Its spreading arms reach out toward the light. It is a hawk that draws its strength from secret springs and rests upon the stone.

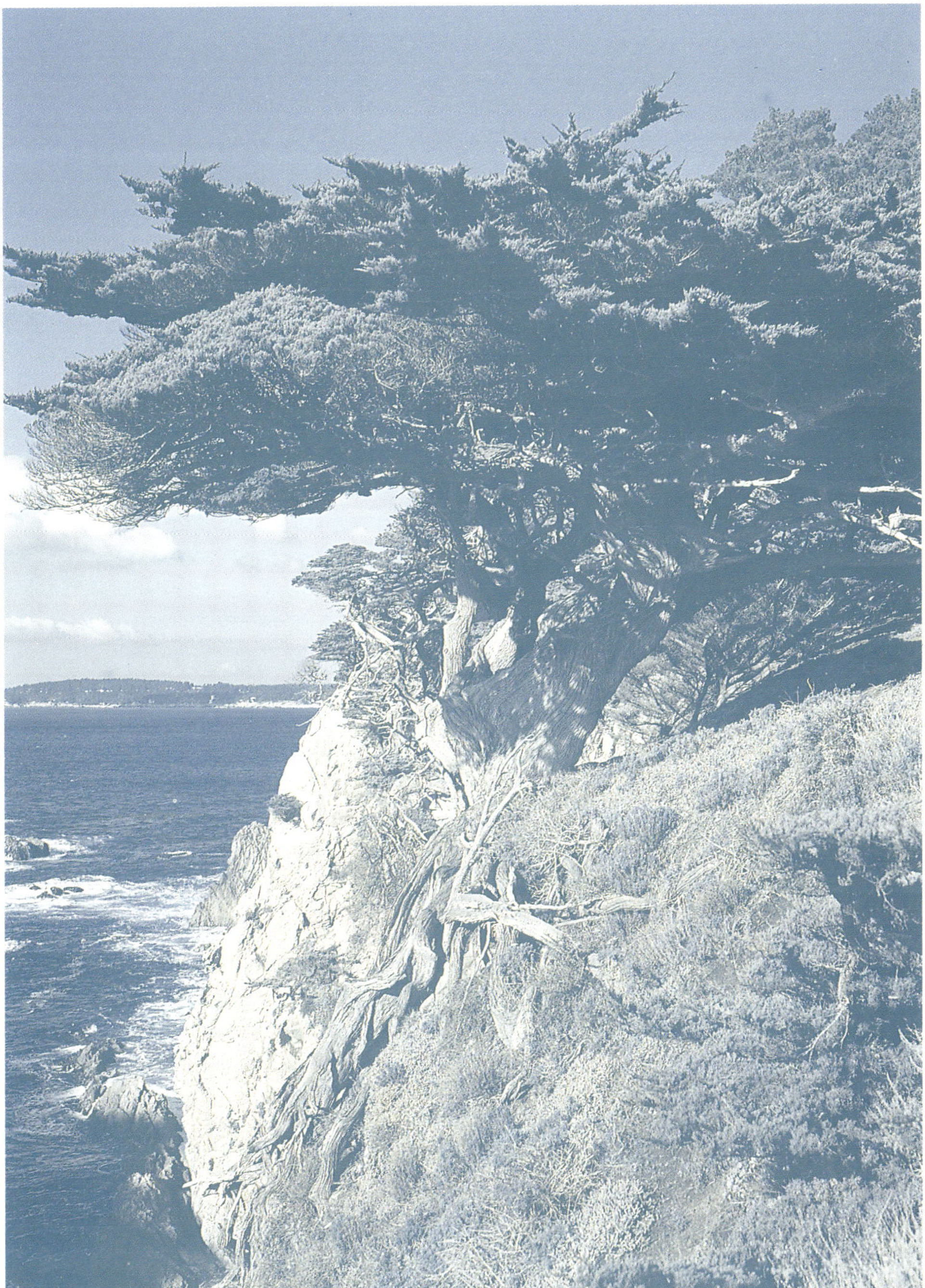

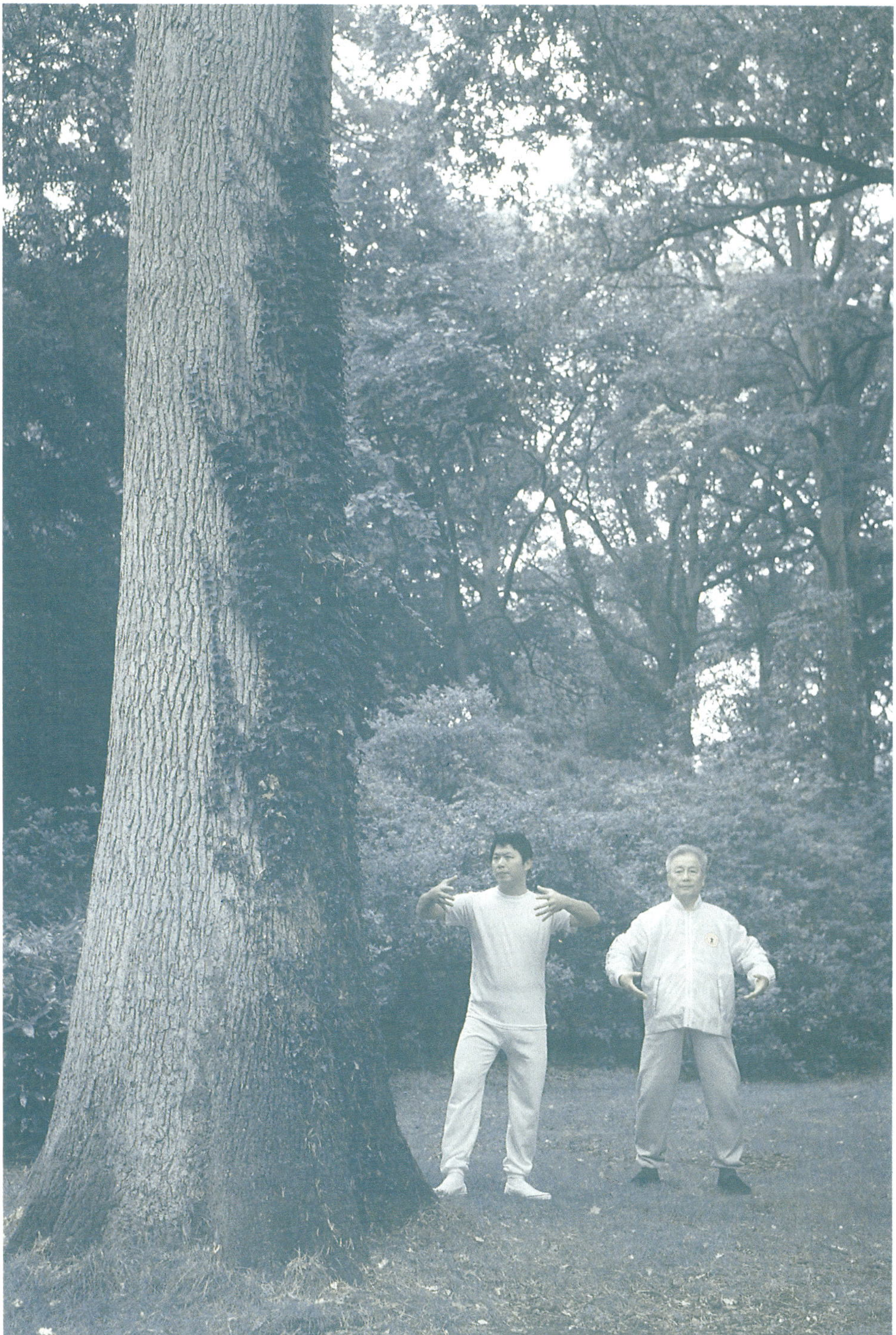

Professor Yu Yong Nian (right) and Master Lam

CHAPTER 7
GOING BEYOND

After about a year of the basic training – the first nine positions – you may feel ready to progress to a higher standard. To many Western people, a year may sound a long time, but if you understand that profound change and growth take time, you will have the patience to continue practising. Remember that you are learning how to realign – and even replace – some of the more distorted and disrupted energy patterns of your life. That sort of radical change cannot be accomplished overnight.

Over your first year of training you should have been aiming to practise standing every day. You have been building up a conditioned response in your body. That takes time and must be activated every day to become automatic. It would not have been surprising if, at the beginning, you had had days when you were tempted to give up. But maybe by the end of the first year (or even the second) you will have found that a period of Zhan Zhuang exercise has become a regular part of your daily life. Even if some days you have very little time to spare, always make sure to fit in even a few minutes of the standing exercises – it is essential not to lose ground. No matter how short a time you spend, you will make some progress every day, growing little by little, like a tree whose growth is imperceptible.

Now is the time to broaden your development by exercising the powers of your mind, as well as the power of your body. In Chapter 2 you learned how to begin to calm your mind. The exercises in this chapter teach you how to focus your energy, so increasing your mental stamina. The more advanced exercises on pages 134 to 136 take you on to a new level of awareness – your quiescent mind starts to become sensitive to the flow of energy both inside your body and in the world around you.

You do not need to practise all of the following exercises at once. Choose which of them you want to do, and fit it (or them) in at the end of your usual Zhan Zhuang practice session, following any additional guidance given with the exercise.

Increasing the powers of your mind

The Balloon Fills with Water

Until now you have been using your mind to help your muscles and nervous system relax while placing your muscles under increasing stress. This exercise takes you in a new direction – it helps to focus the combined energy of your mind and body.

PREPARATION STAGE

Adopt the second position – Holding the Balloon (see p. 35). After you have worked through the basic breathing and relaxing exercises to ensure that your system is calm and centred (see pp. 44-47), apply your mind in a different way.

For 10 to 15 minutes stand quietly, allowing yourself to relax completely. You are holding the imaginary balloon in the embrace of your curved arms.

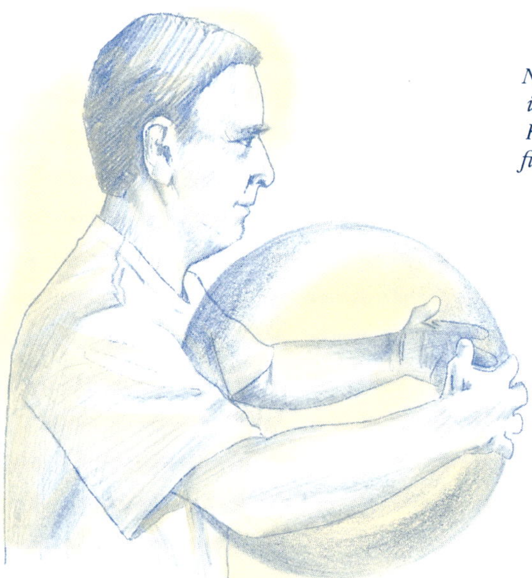

Now imagine that the balloon is slowly filling up with water. Keep holding the balloon as it fills and becomes heavier. Feel the weight of the growing volume of water, but do not move a muscle. If you start to tense up, use your mind to tell your muscles to relax. When the balloon is full, continue standing silently, gently keeping the balloon in place. You will certainly feel the difference created by this mental exercise. Check for any tension in your muscles.

A Hot Shower, a Cold Shower

You can attempt this exercise once you have warmed up and stood for several minutes in the Wu Chi position (see p. 29). It will increase your stamina and help you to use the vitality of your imagination to transcend extreme physical discomfort.

PREPARATION STAGE
After standing in the Wu Chi position for several minutes, move into any one of the other Zhan Zhuang positions.

From the position you have chosen, sink down, remembering not to let your knees come forward over your toes. After a few minutes, you will find you can "sit" even lower. Keep on checking that you have not unconsciously risen upward. Drop down again.

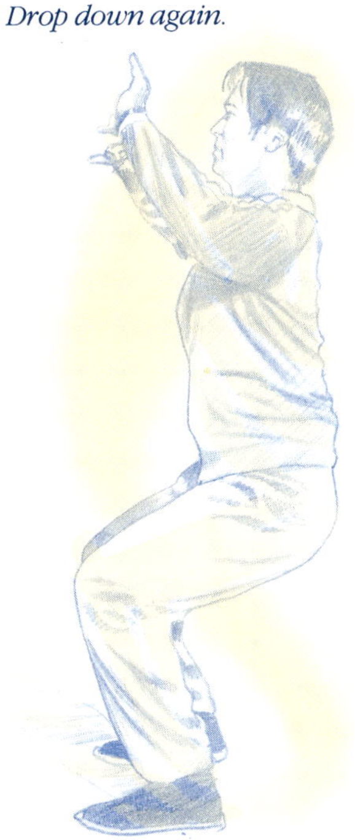

RELAX
After 10 or 15 minutes, make sure that you are completely relaxed from the top of your head to the soles of your feet. This will be difficult, because of the demands you are placing on your legs in your low position. Now is the time for a "shower".

HOT SHOWER
Imagine, without moving, that you are standing under a lovely hot shower. The steaming water is pouring down all over you. As it courses over your body and runs off, it washes your weight and tension away with it. All you can feel is the wonderful stream rushing down your head, torso, arms, and legs. Stand in it, stay low, don't move.

HOLD THE POSITION
As you hold the position you are likely to find that your leg muscles continue to strain. You will probably be sweating, too. Now is the time for a "cold shower".

COLD SHOWER
This is where the extraordinary power of your mind comes in to play again. Imagine that you are standing motionless under a torrent of rushing cold water. It beats on you, pouring over every inch of your flesh. All your sensations are suddenly transformed by the rush of this cold shower. Stand in it, stay low, and try to hold this position for several minutes.

CLOSING POSITION
Slowly rise up and carefully lower your arms. Stand in the Wu Chi position for a minute or two. Shake your arms and legs and walk around slowly.

The Moving Balloon

The fusion of your mind and body reaches a new level with these exercises. The effect on your internal energy is amazing. Now you will begin to understand why it has been so essential to work systematically through the previous stages of your Zhan Zhuang training in order to reach this point.

GROWING PRESSURE

Stand in the second position – Holding the Balloon (see p. 35). After you feel comfortable in this position, make sure your fingers are held open so that you can imagine holding little balls or marbles between them.

Imagine that the balloon is pressing outward on your hands, as if trying to escape from your embrace. Now use your mind to keep your hands in place, resisting the growing pressure of the balloon. Do not tense up.

Now the balloon tries to push out the opposite way, through your chest. Use the power of your mind to allow your chest to hold the balloon in place.

Now the balloon presses to the right, against your right forearm and elbow. Again, your mind prevents it from escaping. It tries your left forearm and elbow. Your mind stops it pressing past your arm.

The balloon tries to escape upward. Your mind is suddenly present in your thumbs and holds it in place. The balloon tries to escape downward. Your little fingers prevent it.

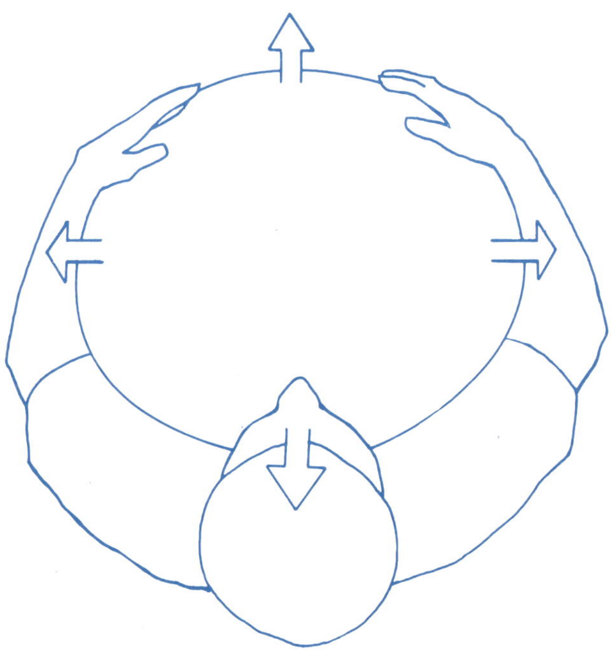

Now the balloon tries to escape in different and opposite directions at the same time, eventually trying to break out of your embrace by expanding outward simultaneously in all six directions. Your mind must work ceaselessly to keep the balloon in place.

THE PULL OF MAGNETS
Now imagine that you are surrounded by magnets that gently attract your arms and torso at various points. Two attract the backs of your hands, pulling them slightly outward. Two attract your elbows, drawing them to either side. One exerts a pull on the middle of your back (see below). The force of these magnets is not as strong as the expanding force of the balloon that you are trying to hold in place, but you can feel in your mind the pull they are exerting.

Do not allow your mind to rest. Feel the constant movement and pressure of the balloon; feel the gentle pull of the magnets. On the outside, nothing is moving. Everything is taking place within you.

Sink back on your heels for a minute or two – or longer if you can – and lower your bottom, gripping the floor with your toes to keep from falling backward.

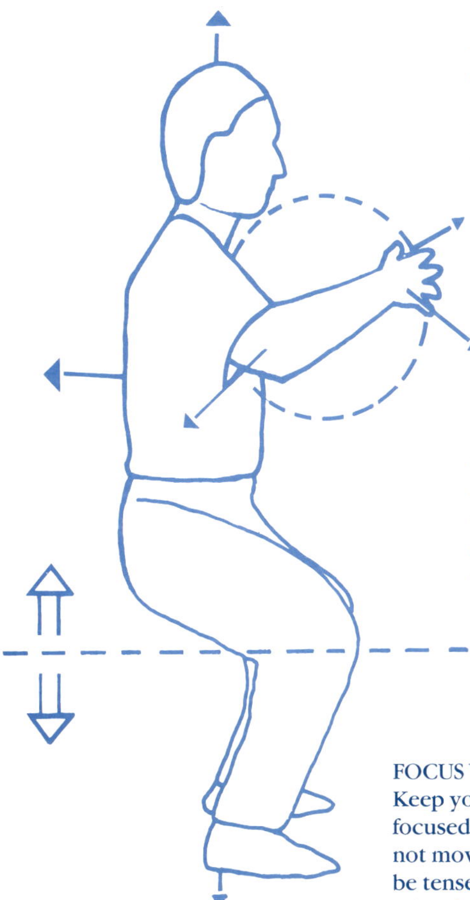

As you hold this extreme position and your mind is wholly engaged by the escaping balloon, imagine that your heels extend downward with maximum force into the centre of the earth. The top of your head is drawn upward at the same time into space. You are suspended between space and earth. Your back is drawn backward by an infinitely distant and powerful force. All that keeps you from being sucked backward is an equal force pulling the back of your hands; holding you in place.

FOCUS YOUR MIND
Keep your mind utterly focused on these forces. Do not move. No muscle should be tense. You are held in the grip of powerful forces, but like a tree you are unmoved. You may only be able to hold this position for a few minutes, but they may pass surprisingly quickly, as your normal sense of time can be distorted during this exercise.

Going beyond

The mind in action

The powerful effect of the "mentality exercises" described in Chapter 2 and The Balloon Fills with Water, and A Hot Shower, A Cold Shower, will have already shown you the indispensable role of the mind in the Zhan Zhuang system. If possible take the advice of an instructor before advancing to this next stage. Do not attempt this level unless you are able to stand comfortably in the nine Zhan Zhuang postures for the recommended period of time.

This is an extraordinarily intense exercise. Your pulse and body heat will shoot up, but your breathing will remain calm and deep. Inside your body, a violent thunderstorm will be under way, but you will appear calm and unmoving. Build up gradually, working on one or two sets of muscles in each training session.

TENSE AND RELAX

Adopt the second position – Holding the Balloon (see p. 35). Hold it for 15 minutes and relax both your body and your mind (see Chapter 2). Then use your mind to tense and relax specific muscle groups systematically.

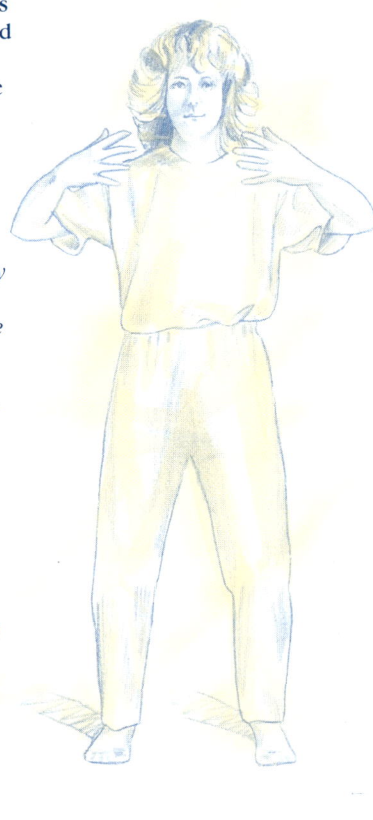

Begin with your left calf muscle. Tense it. Relax it. Do this 30 times. Don't move any other muscles. If they move, relax them. Then do the same with your right calf muscle. Then move on to your left thigh muscle, then your right thigh muscle, and then the muscle in your left buttock. Finally, tense the muscle in your right buttock.

Now tense larger groups of muscles 30 times each. First tense your whole left leg and buttock and relax. Then do the same for your right leg and buttock.

Move then to your arms. Tense your left hand, then your right hand, your left forearm, your right forearm, your left upper arm, and your right upper arm, 30 times each.

Then tense and relax your entire left arm and then your right arm 30 times each.

Finish by tensing both legs and buttocks together 30 times, then both arms and hands 30 times, then your arms and legs 30 times.

Do not tense your torso or your neck.

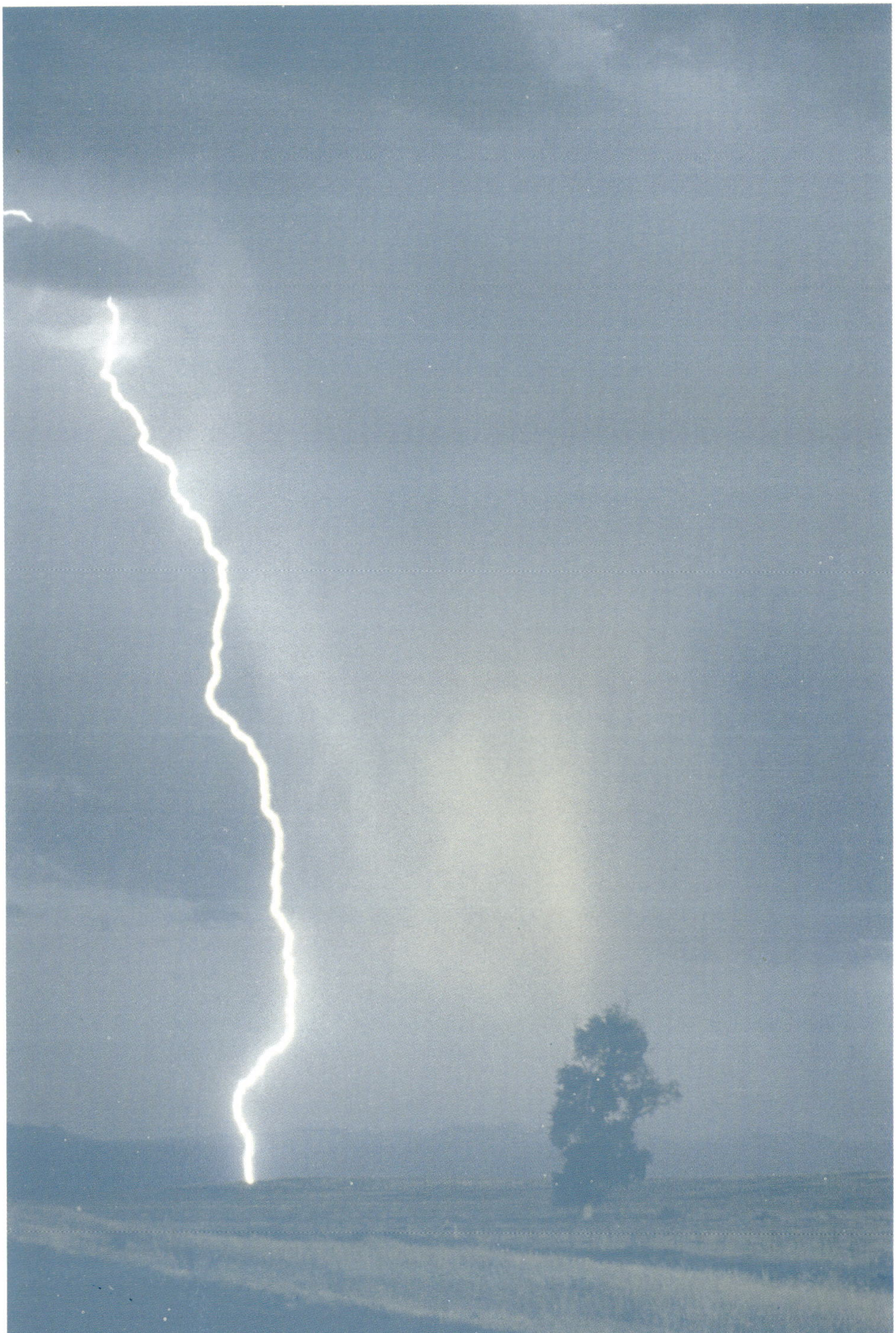

Using imagery

The following exercise assumes that you have managed to perform the initial mental relaxation exercises described in Chapter 2. It takes you beyond conventional thinking, and aims to achieve a perfectly quiescent mind. The inner commotion and noisy activity of your mind (the usual stream of memories, inner dialogue, and mental anxiety) is stilled and your mind becomes extraordinarily sensitive and alert. Reaching this stage is one of the hardest things for any human being to do. You are changing the fundamental behaviour of your mind: it will be doing absolutely nothing.

PREPARATION STAGE

Begin by standing in one of the Zhan Zhuang positions. In the beginning, you will find it easiest to adopt the first or second position. You will probably find the second position – Holding the Balloon (see p. 35) best as the basis for this advanced work on the mind. At this level, you should not worry about your breathing. You are going beyond that stage and returning, full circle, to your original state.

BE TRANQUIL

Check that your muscle groups are relaxed throughout your body. Even after several years' practice you may find that your relaxation is still superficial. Deep layers of solidified anxiety and nervous strain have accumulated over the years. You may be only now beginning to get in touch with those tensions and you may start to feel strange sensations as they begin to melt. Just as at the beginning of your training, you may experience unexpected heat, cold, sweating, and abrupt shaking.

As you relax further your body comes to rest. Your nervous system relaxes. You reach the state of tranquillity that you have become familiar with from the mentality exercises described earlier, in Chapter 2.

EXTEND YOUR PRACTICE

If you have not reached this stage in your training, the passages that follow on pages 132 and 133 can, inevitably, remain only words on the page. Just continue patiently with your standing: every day you are growing within. One day these words will open beautifully before you like blossoms.

If you sense that you are ready for this stage of training, treat each of the following passages as a direction for the further extension of your practice. These are not mantras or texts for recitation or meditation. Nor are they instructions or guided imagery. When you have reached this level of Zhan Zhuang, they will simply be companions on your way.

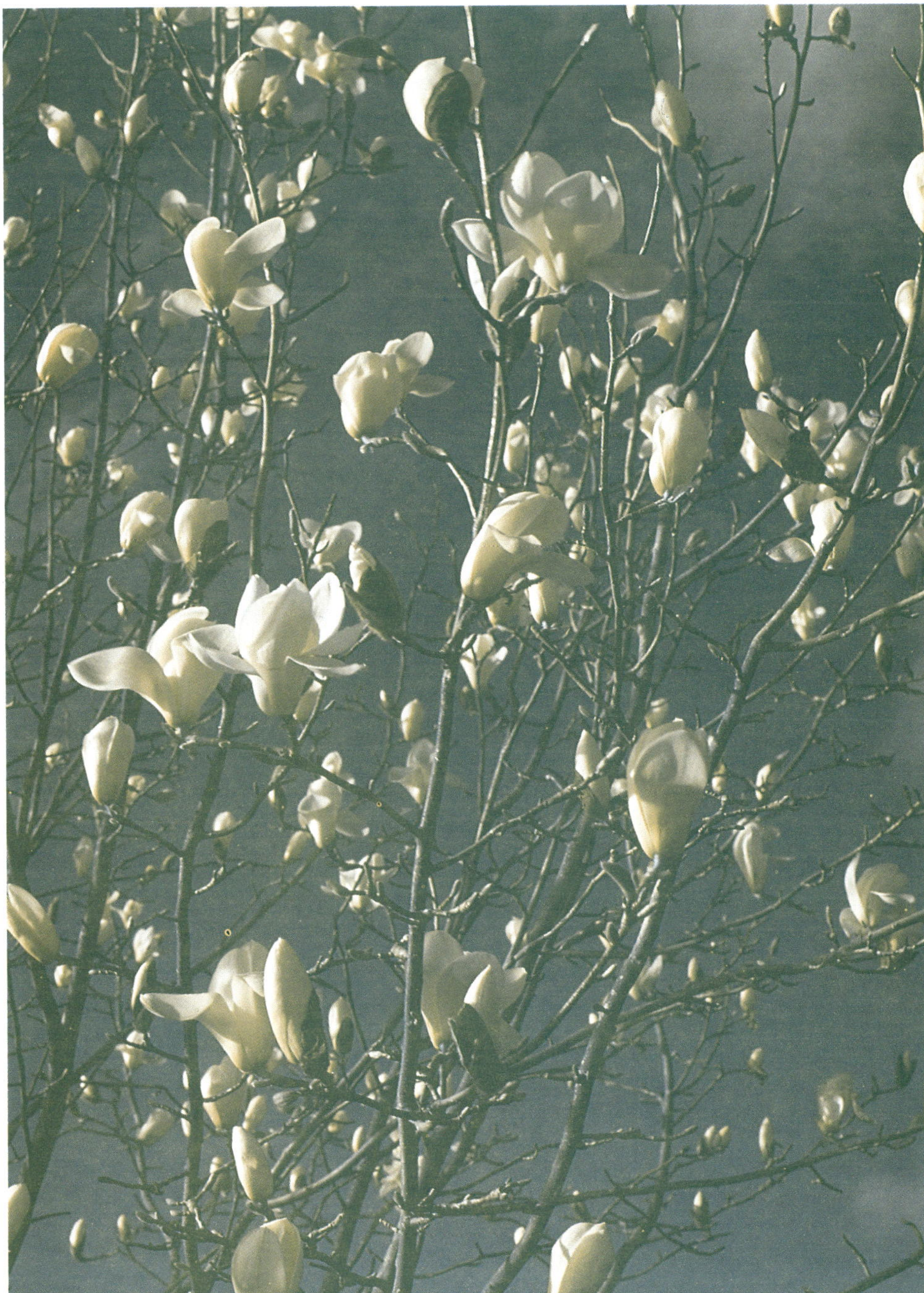

Standing like a tree

You are standing like a tree. You are like an elm growing. You feel everything happening within your entire body, from your roots deep in the soil, to the tiniest leaf reaching out into the air. You can hear yourself moving inside. You are growing, listening silently to your entire body inhaling and exhaling.

A living tree breathes with its entire body. Every cell of every leaf is breathing. Deep in the earth, the roots are breathing too. As you stand, you do the same. Open every pore of your body – along your arms, down your back and legs, from the soles of your feet to the top of your head. Feel the lovely breeze entering inside you at every conceivable point of your being. And as you exhale, let the warm current ride out again from every extremity.

You stand surrounded, like a tree, by sound. All noise within is stilled. Sounds come to you, as if from miles around. Birds call from distant tree tops. An engine starts up somewhere far away. Here and there you hear a footfall and a man and woman with a child. Nearby you hear the early morning drone of an insect. The air around you is alive. Can you hear the dew drops falling in the grass?

You stand, seeing a tree in the distance. There is nothing but empty space between the tree and you. You are both silent. Your eyes are completely at peace and a faint smile is all you sense. Your body is asleep. Your mind is alert.

A distant wind is stirring in the air. It starts to play across your body like a flag unfurling in a breeze. The driving air is irresistible; the flag is flying with it. All seems to be in motion, but neither sky nor flag has moved.

A fish is turning in the stream. Its weight is in the water; the fish itself is still. Like you, it rests inside the current. Its body curves a little and it sways. It does not matter that the wind has made the surface rough.

Your boat is on the waves. The tide is strong: it pulls and twists the boat from side to side. You stand within it, riding in the surge. You tremble for a moment, but you do not leave the boat. You know the water knows its way.

The wind is rising and the storm clouds threaten rain. You stand among the trees, like them, unmoved. They all have stood in sun and shade. Their roots have been both dry and wet. Now rain and wind will fill the sky. The trees, like you, have no wish to escape. Like you, they stand prepared to feel the deepest movements of the earth.

New awareness

Feeling the energy flow

As you make progress in your Zhan Zhuang training you will become sensitive not only to the remarkable flow of energy inside you, but also to the energy that surrounds you. The exercises that follow enhance your sensitivity to this energy in nature. The two circuits that are described below correspond to internal energy pathways in your own system. You will start to feel the marvellous effect of linking these with the internal power of trees and flowering bushes.

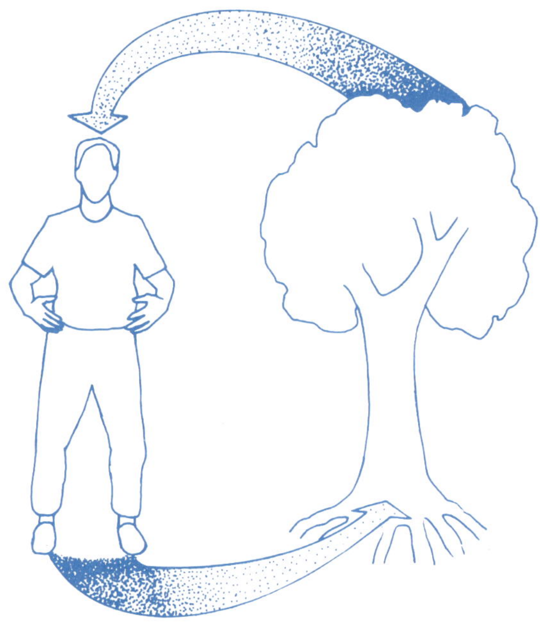

PREPARATION STAGE

A very advanced exercise starts by standing near a large tree, at any time of the year. Complete the full warm up exercises, including the advanced level of Ba Duan Jin. Then begin standing in any of the Zhan Zhuang positions; the most commonly used is Holding the Balloon – the second position (see p. 35). Allow your system to calm down and become thoroughly relaxed. This involves achieving both physical and mental quiescence (see pp. 44-47). Stand quietly.

HOLD THE POSITION

If you are used to holding the basic standing positions for 20 minutes or longer, you will probably find that you can maintain this variation for the same length of time.

As you stand, allow the tree to become the sole object of your attentive mind. Imagine that there is a circuit of energy that extends from the top of your head to the crown of the spreading tree. Imagine that the circuit is completed between the soles of your feet and the roots of the tree in the earth. There is now a full cycle of natural energy flowing through both of you. You become part of the tree. There is one circuit, one field of energy: the fused, identical power of the tree and you.

As the energy flows in from above, breathe in to draw the Chi deeply into yourself. Exhale as the energy flows out from your feet into the ground.

SECOND CIRCUIT
The next stage in this exercise begins by facing the tree. Stand in the second position – Holding the Balloon (see p. 35).

You will gain the maximum benefit from these exercises if you stand in front of a particularly strong tree. It is not by accident that so many Chinese landscape paintings portray evergreens. Their Chi is particularly powerful, which makes them ideal for these exercises.

In summer try standing before a strong, flowering bush. The effect is wondrous, particularly in the early morning.

PREPARATION STAGE
Open your hands outward, as if embracing the air in front of you. The fingers of both hands should be pointing gently toward the tree.

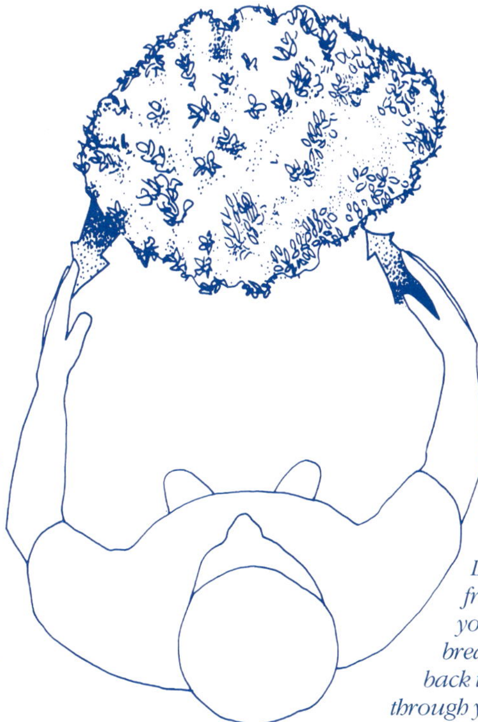

Now open a new circuit of energy. Draw in the Chi from the tree through your left hand as you breathe in. Circle it back to the tree out through your right hand as you exhale (see left).

"When I stand," said Wang Xiang Zhai, "the earth is in my hands. The universe is in my mind."

"You are free," he told his students. "You are a great fire. If anything comes toward you, it will be consumed in the fire. If it does not approach the fire, it will not be burned. You are merely the fire. You remain where you are, content to be alight."

"You are the sea. Whatever anyone gives you, you can take. They can also take from you anything they want. The sea is vast; it can give up anything and still remain the sea. Like the sea, you are endless and unceasing. This is the true freedom."

Energy from the galaxy

There is a level of higher training that may interest some readers. It can be reached only after long, dedicated practice.

The exercises on pages 124 to 135 will have increased the power of your mind. The exercise that follows makes great demands on that power and stretches your mind into the solar system.

The ideal time for this exercise is sunrise. Stand facing the rising sun. Let it be the destination for your orbiting energy and bring back into yourself the power of its rays.

FOCUS YOUR ENERGY
Stand in the second position – Holding the Balloon (see p. 35). Focus all your attention on your navel. Imagine that your energy has become a little point, a small satellite ready to go into orbit around you. It makes a single circle around your waist, moving anticlockwise. It travels at a gentle, natural pace and is ready to begin a second circuit around you, this time just a little further away from your body. As it travels around you, your body may sway a little; this is natural, but don't mistake this slight physical movement for the real point of the exercise, which is the circulation of the energy around you.

WIDENING CIRCLES
Keep the point of energy rotating around you in ever-widening circles. They begin to reach far beyond the place where you are standing: beyond your room; beyond the park; beyond your town; beyond your country; beyond your continent – circling as wide as the earth and then spinning into space.

21 ORBITS
Make 21 orbits, reaching the sun or the moon on the 21st. Pause for one or two seconds. Then begin the return journey, this time circling back in clockwise loops until the travelling point of energy returns to your navel, on the 21st of these ever-diminishing clockwise orbits.

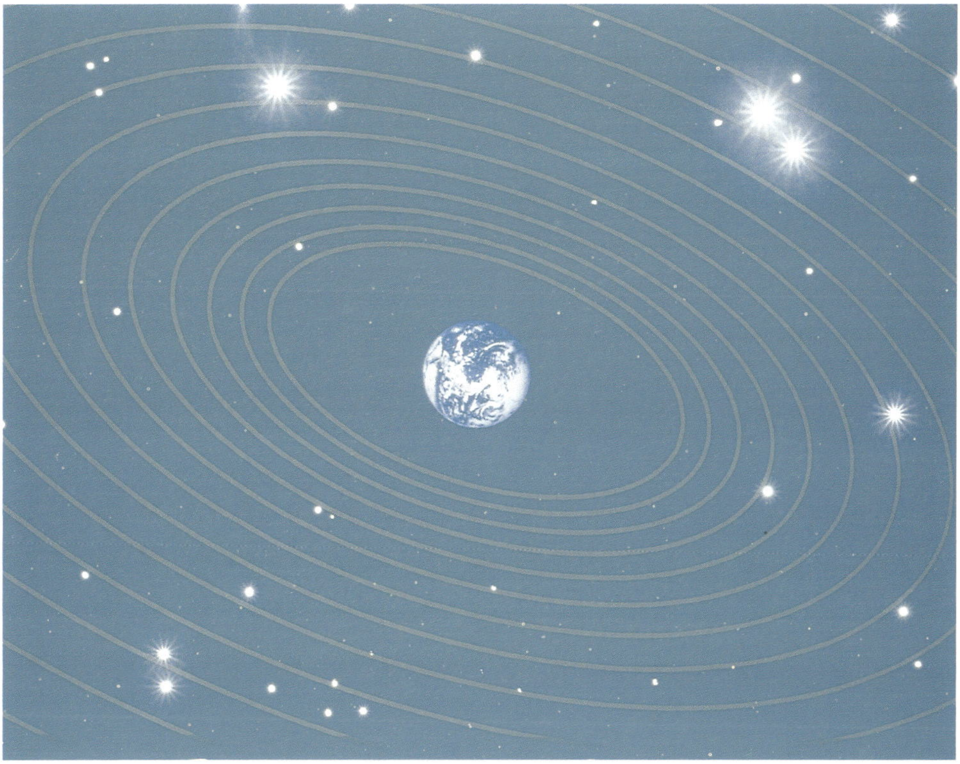

"Non-action is the real action.
One hundred acts are not as good as one moment of silence.
One hundred exercises are not as good as one moment of standing still."

"Big action is not as good as small action.
Small action is not as good as non-action."

Wang Xiang Zhai

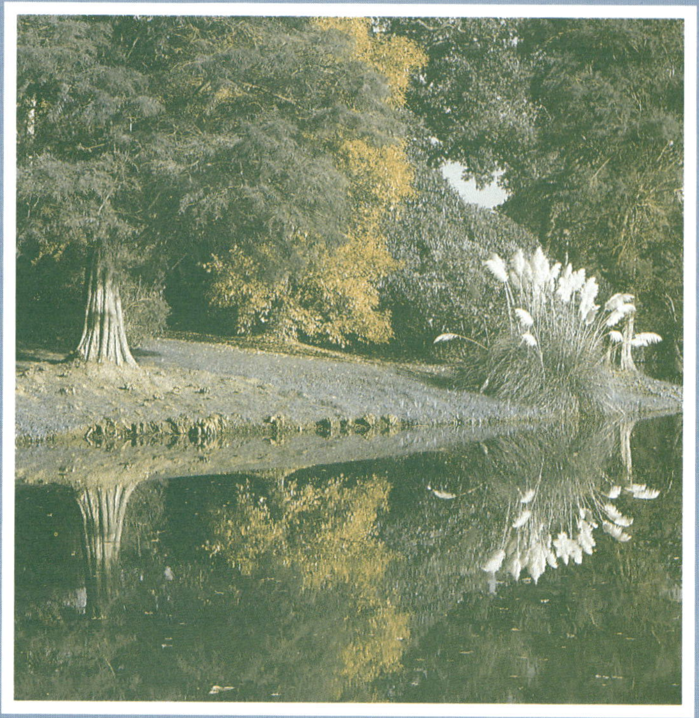

PART FOUR

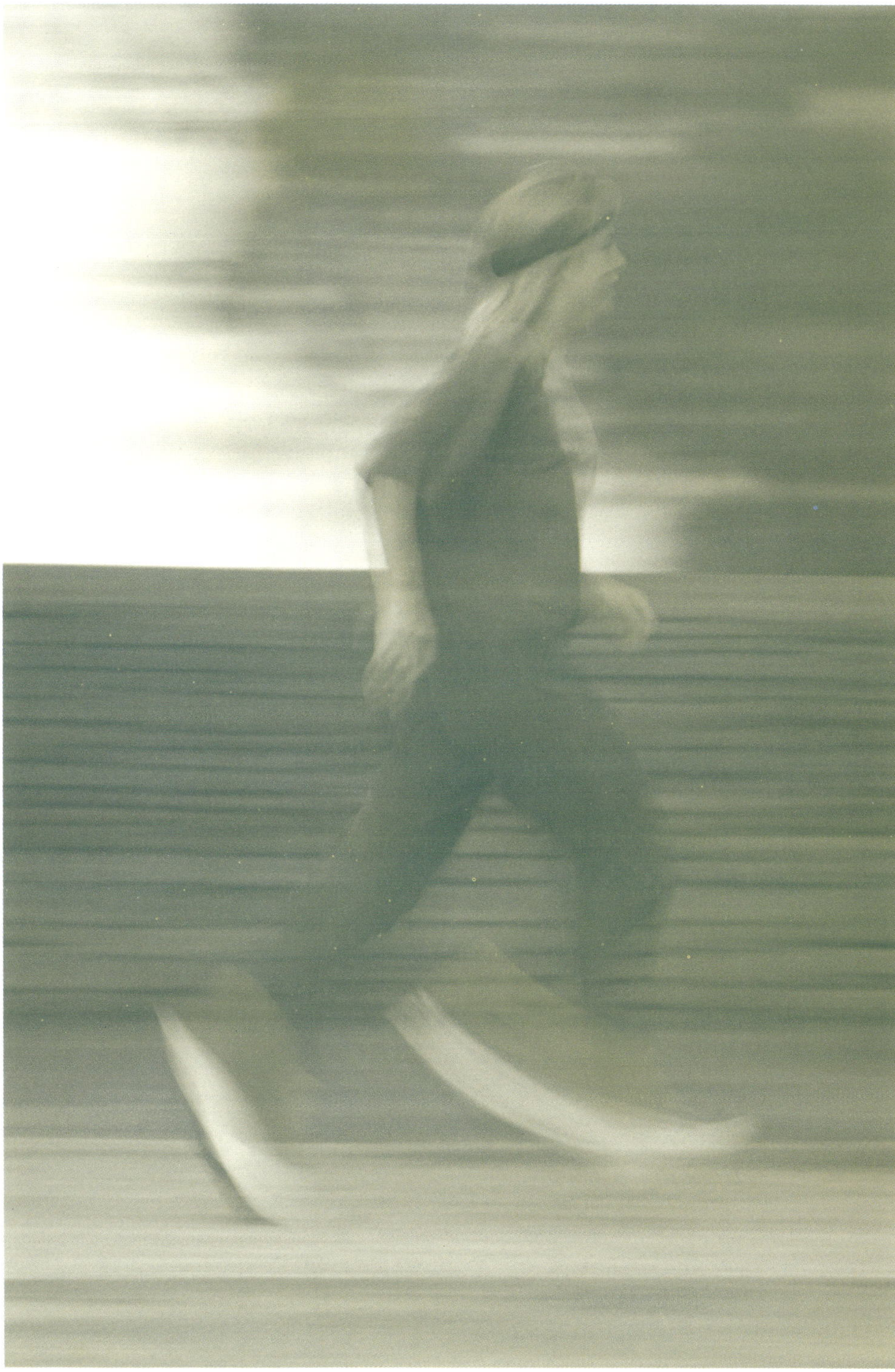

CHAPTER 8
ENERGY IN DAILY LIFE

Energy is always circulating throughout your body. It permeates all living tissue and all organ systems. But the pressures of your day-to-day life, the physical hassles and mental stresses, can cause energy to stagnate. It can become blocked and, over time, cease to flow to vital organs. Tense, contracted muscles produce stiff and abrupt movements that block the natural, sustained flow of your energy. These hard, hasty movements ultimately slow you down because they inhibit and then exhaust your energy. By contrast, gentle rhythmic movement can be continued with greater effect over much longer periods of time.

There are numerous moments in the day, whether at home, travelling, at work, or even while sleeping, when you can apply the basic principles of the Zhan Zhuang exercises. They will not only help you relax, but will also help you freshen up and concentrate with renewed vigour. There are even ways you can do a little exercise so discreetly that no one will realize it.

All you have to do is to apply the Zhan Zhuang postures you have already learned to the situations you find yourself in each day. This will ease the pathways of your internal energy, making your movements more fluid, less prone to accident, more balanced, and less tiring.

You can also reduce the tension in your body during everyday activities by paying attention to how you do things. When you brush your teeth, do you exert a lot of pressure on the toothbrush? Is your wrist stiff? When you write, do you press down hard with your pen or pencil? Are your arm muscles tense? When you use a paintbrush, saw, or scrubbing brush, is your grip stronger than you need to do the job smoothly?

The great Chinese calligraphers take up their writing brushes with a minimum of effort and produce faultless flowing movements that are at the same time full of vigour and completely controlled. Try this when you hold a cup, take a photograph, or polish the kitchen table, for example, and you will get the same effect with less muscle pressure.

The daily cycle

You can practise your Zhan Zhuang training at any time in the day by adapting the positions to suit your daily activities. For example, you can practise the second position – Holding the Balloon – while sitting in the office (page 146), when travelling (page 150), or while watching television (page 152). Even practising for a few minutes will be refreshing, and the effect will intensify as you build up your Zhan Zhuang practice every day.

From the moment you get out of bed in the morning and through your day, you can use your Zhan Zhuang training to improve your performance. Even when you go to sleep, the positions on the facing page will help you.

GETTING UP

First thing in the morning, even if you are not fully awake, stand quietly beside your bed. Stand in a comfortable, natural position, with your hands hanging loosely by your sides, for two or three minutes. Don't stand longer than five minutes. Just relax with your eyes open or closed, whichever you find most comfortable. After that you can start your normal morning activities. If you need to use the toilet the very first thing in the morning, do that before standing, but don't do things like washing your face or brushing your teeth, which jar your system awake. Do those only after you have been standing still for a few minutes.

Sitting, holding the balloon

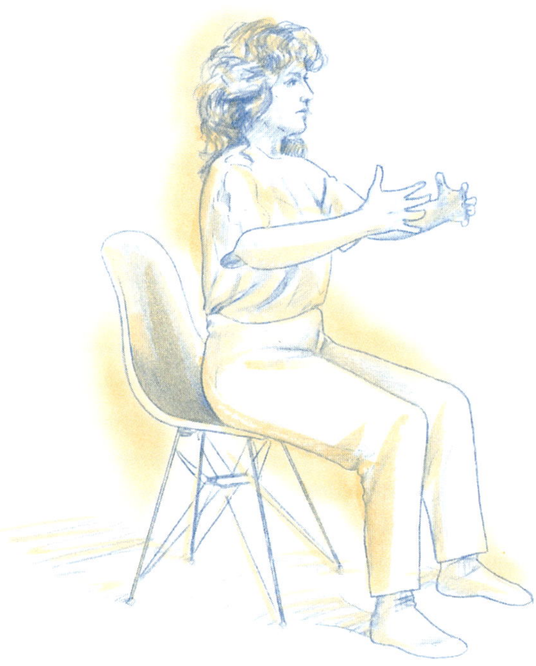

STANDING AND SITTING

Remember that whenever you are standing or sitting, you can find a way to relax and practise your exercises at the same time. For example, when sitting, don't slouch against the back of the chair. Sit slightly away from the back, rest your forearms on the armrests, or rest your wrists on your thighs. Open your hands slightly as if holding an invisible balloon in your lap. Or rest your forearms and open hands on the table in front of you.

SLEEPING

We are seldom fully relaxed when asleep. Even without nightmares, our sleep is disturbed by latent tensions and we are often in constant, fitful movement. Try to calm yourself and centre your energy around your navel before you sleep, by using any of the three positions illustrated below.

1. Lie on your right side, so as not to put pressure on your heart. Slide your left knee over your right thigh. Put your right hand under your right cheek and your left hand on top of your left hip.

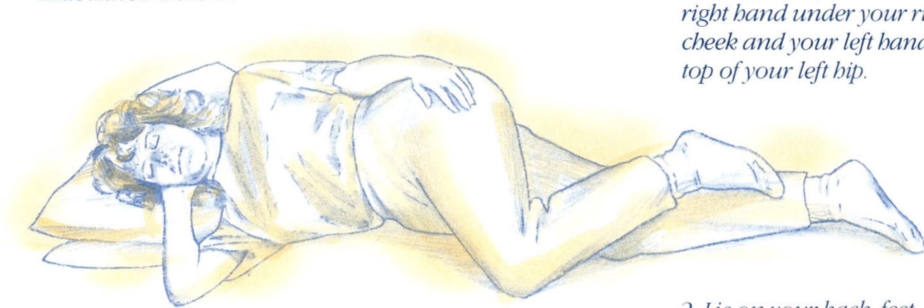

2. Lie on your back, feet slightly apart. Rest your hands, palms down, on your belly.

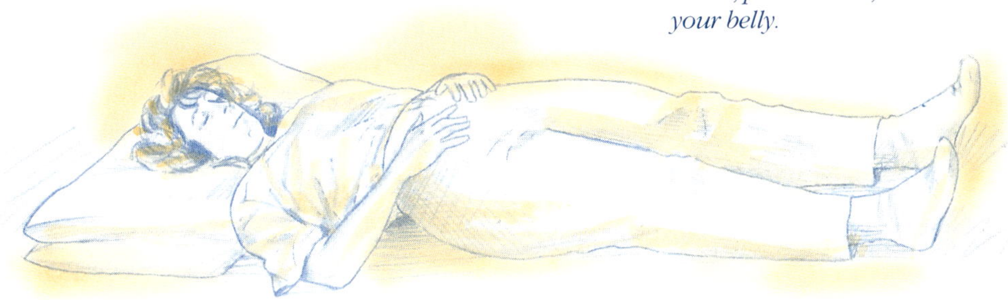

3. Lie on your back, feet slightly apart. Rest your hands, palms down, beside you.

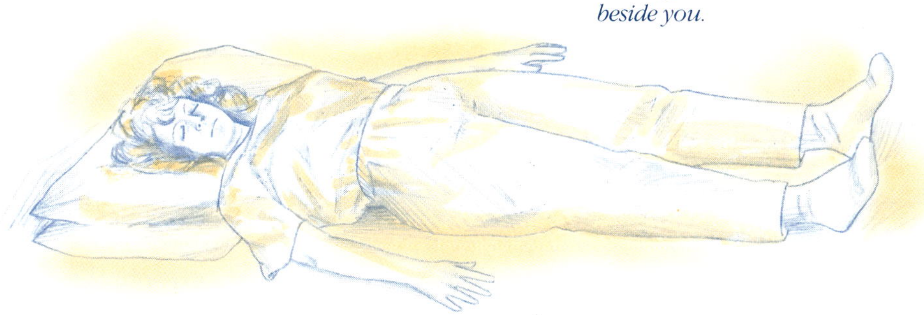

Domestic work

When washing up, dusting, vacuuming, making beds, or doing any other tasks around the home, look carefully at what you are doing. Are you gripping things so tightly that your knuckles go white? Are you tensing all the muscles in your arms and neck? Are you twisting your spine into awkward positions? Any time you find yourself doing these things, stop. Straighten up. Let the tension drain away from your muscles and then see if you can use the basic principles of Zhan Zhuang to accomplish the task, with minimum muscle and maximum energy.

While out shopping, too, you will have lots of opportunities to practise Zhan Zhuang and to put its principles into effect.

As you walk, drive, or go by public transport to the market or shops, use the techniques described on pages 150 to 51 to develop your ability to relax.

OUT SHOPPING

When lifting and carrying, remember to use your energy, not your muscle. See how lightly you can grasp and hold things without dropping them – you will quickly see how much unnecessary muscular force and tension you waste on daily tasks.

When you are carrying a basket, or reaching for items, or just moving around in a shop, pay attention to your shoulders. Are they nicely relaxed – or are they hunched up from force of habit?

If you are pushing a shopping cart in a supermarket, don't use a tight grip. Let your hands or wrists rest on it. Your weight will naturally move it forward. Experiment with it when you turn it. Are you gripping it and filling your arms and shoulders with tension, or are you guiding it like a balloon, with a light upper body and your feet firmly rooted beneath you?

While you wait to pay, don't miss the opportunity for a little discreet Zhan Zhuang exercise. After all, you are standing, so practise any of the standing exercises you feel are appropriate and make invaluable use of your time!

ARTHRITIS TIP

A mistake quite a few people make is to plunge their hands among the boxes of frozen food, often unnecessarily. Even doing this once a week can contribute to arthritic complaints. Whenever possible, look to see what you want, then quickly pick it up and put it straight into your basket.

DON'T SLUMP

When you want to take a break from household chores, or if you feel exhausted when you get home from shopping, don't just throw yourself down on a sofa. That is bad for your posture, bad for your breathing, and bad for your energy. Take a few minutes to renew your energy and refresh yourself with a little Zhan Zhuang. You'll be amazed at how good you feel.

Sit or stand in one of the Zhan Zhuang positions for several minutes. Start relaxing from the top of your head, down through your neck, shoulders, and spine, and down to your feet. The tension caused by heavy use of your muscles will ease and the natural circulation of vital energy will happen on its own.

You can also give yourself an "energy wash" (see right).

CALM YOUR ANGER

If you allow yourself to become angry or tense, the flow of energy in your body can get seriously blocked. Zhan Zhuang will help you calm down. Whatever you are doing, stop. Pour a glass of water. If possible, use a light green glass, as the colour green has a powerful calming effect on the nervous system. Set the glass of water down in front of you. Then stand or sit, holding your arms in any of the basic Zhan Zhuang positions. While in the position, gaze at the water in the glass. The Chinese way is to gaze at an aquarium to calm the spirit. Within minutes you will feel the natural balance and inner strength of your system being restored.

ENERGY WASH

When you are at home or at work and you are getting tired, or becoming tense and angry, you can use your natural energy reserves to restore your vitality and calm your nerves.

When you feel tired, go and wash your face in warm water and dry it. Then sit down at a desk or table. Put your hands and forearms on the table, and hold your hands loosely open, holding the invisible balloon. Close your eyes. Breathe naturally, calmly, and quietly. Sit still in that position for two to three minutes. Then open your eyes. Lift your hands and "wash" your face several times with your palms, moving slowly up from your chin, over your face, and back across your ears. This will rapidly refresh your system at any time of the day and recharge the energy of your body and mind. You can also do it in one of the Zhan Zhuang standing positions, the second position is probably the best.

At work

Many people damage their backs and wear themselves out by regularly sitting in hunched, cramped, and stressful positions at their desks and in meetings. Ask yourself: do you often push your shoulders up by leaning forward heavily on your elbows? Do you twist your spine and cross your legs? Do you curve downward in a slouch as you sit? Do you compress your chest by folding your arms in various ways?

We unthinkingly generate a lot of physical stress in our bodies during our working day. Even the most basic office practices such as answering the telephone or making a call are likely to create tension. But you can convert telephone calls, and many of your work movements, into excellent short Zhan Zhuang practice sessions, which free your energy and leave you more alert for your work.

Breaking the bad habits of a lifetime won't be easy. Whenever you catch yourself holding tension in your body, try to incorporate a little Zhan Zhuang exercise into whatever you are doing.

SITTING

Move slightly forward in your chair so your back is completely free. Slowly straighten your back. Don't arch it, just let it straighten naturally. Place both feet flat on the floor. Don't cross your legs, especially over your thighs, as this restricts the flow in some of your major arteries. Rest your forearms on the armrests of your chair; or rest your wrists on your thighs. Keep your upper arms away from your torso, leaving your chest free to move.

At a desk or table, rest your forearms (not your elbows) on the surface, with your weight dropping downward on your hanging elbows – not pressing upward into your neck and shoulders.

Let your hands curve naturally and think of holding a large balloon gently between them. Breathe naturally and quietly. Keep your mind on what you are reading or saying or listening to. Your relaxed body will keep your mind alert.

Adapt the second position as shown below when working at your desk.

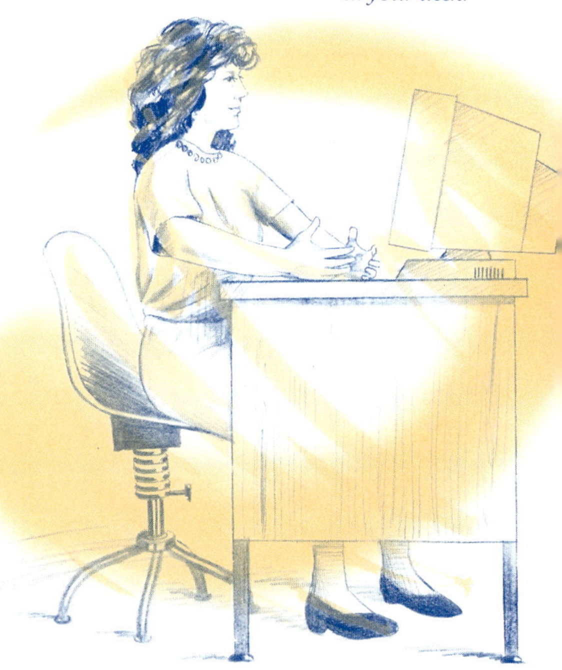

ON THE TELEPHONE

If you are standing when you use the phone, shift your weight on to one leg. Angle your other foot slightly away. Hold the receiver lightly with only the thumb and first fingers of the hand on the side of your body that is bearing your weight. Relax your other fingers, your wrist, and your forearm. There should be no tension in your torso or the side of your body that is not bearing your weight.

If you are seated, lean your upper body weight on the elbow of the arm you are using to hold the phone. Shift your weight to that side of your body so that it runs down through your elbow, your buttock, and your foot. The other side of your body should feel completely weightless. Hold the receiver lightly using only your thumb and first finger.

Hold your head upright and relax the free side of your body as you hold the phone.

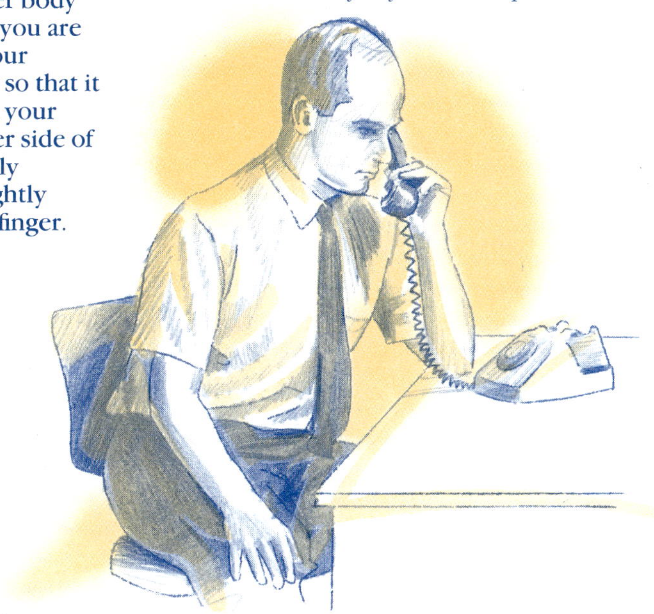

DO NOT:

- hold the receiver by hunching up your shoulder

- lean your head over to one side while talking: keep it upright

- grip the receiver: hold it lightly

- fold your free arm across your chest and tuck it under your other arm – this constricts your chest

At the computer

The problems caused by working at a computer keyboard are similar to the results of prolonged typing, writing, or playing the piano. The underlying cause is tension and in extreme cases, the strain leads to damage of the nerves in the wrist. In traditional Chinese medicine, the condition is cured by massage, the application of herbs, and special exercises.

You can use the Chi Kung technique described below to help prevent or relieve tension and pain in the hands. Do the exercise for a few minutes before starting work at the keyboard or if you start to feel tired while working.

FINGER EXERCISES

Stand in the second position – Holding the Balloon (see pp. 34-35) for two or three minutes. Then, lower your hands to elbow height, loosely outstretched and facing downward in front of you, as if resting on a counter. Follow the instructions (below, right), then massage your hands all over.

If you are seated, you can do the same thing in the sitting position, making sure your back is naturally vertical and not curled against the back of your chair.

These finger exercises not only help to remove the strain in your hands and improve the circulation of blood in your fingers, but are also excellent stimulation for your brain.

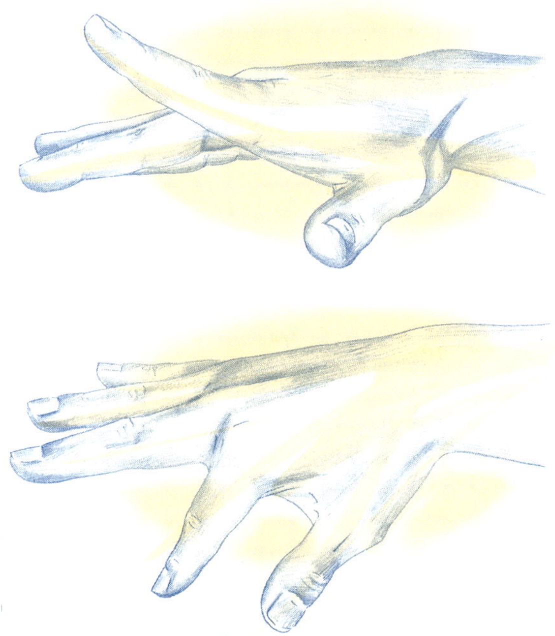

Slowly raise both thumbs, trying not to move your other fingers. Hold for one second. Then lower them, pressing down as far as you can for one second, keeping your other fingers still. Relax your thumbs and repeat for each of your other pairs of fingers. Do the whole set slowly and smoothly several times.

TAKE A BREAK

Some people are mesmerized by computer screens and work for hours without a break. This is the cause of many stress-induced complaints, such as eye strain, tension in the back, and headaches. Look after yourself: take a break at least once an hour. Get up, walk around and do something else for a few minutes before resuming work. This is essential if you want to avoid long-term problems.

The dentist, the bricklayer, and the wallpaper hanger

Three people I know well use Zhan Zhuang in their work. One is a young bricklayer. He has started using gentle, rhythmic movements while he lays down the mortar and places the bricks. He tells me that since becoming a student of Zhan Zhuang, he is able to keep at this strenuous work without getting tired, and he has far fewer accidents.

Another student, an older man, is a wallpaper hanger. He tells me he has developed a set of easy, flowing gestures for brushing the paste on the wall, gently positioning the paper, and smoothing it into place. He says, "The young men with me hang five panels and then they need a break. They're all tired. I carry on working and can easily do up to ten panels at a time. It's fantastic: I just do one after another... the flow never stops."

My master, Yu Yong Nian, is a professor of dentistry in Beijing. He uses his Zhan Zhuang exercises to help him in his professional life. Usually when dentists pull teeth, they have to struggle as they pull hard on the teeth with their pliers. My master administers the local anaesthetic, does his Zhan Zhuang standing exercise for two or three minutes, and then pops the patient's tooth out in a single, flowing gesture. He can work 10 to 12 hours a day. I know no one else who can work with the same power.

Travelling

Think of all the ways that most of us move about in our daily lives – on foot, on public transport, in cars. Each of these modes of transport provides opportunities for some discreet Zhan Zhuang practice, whether it be a moment of relaxation or a modified posture for standing or sitting.

On public transport

WAITING

Stand in the first position – the Wu Chi posture (see p. 29). Your whole body is relaxed. Shift your full weight on to one leg. Turn your other leg outward at a slight angle. Slip your hands inside your pockets, leaving only your thumbs outside. Rest the full weight of your hands on your pockets. Feel your shoulders sinking downward. Breathe naturally. When you tire of one position, shift your weight to your other leg, or on to both feet equally. Feel free to look around and to talk, but try to keep the rest of your body completely still.

If you have no pockets: stand in the first position, weight on one leg or on both feet. Hold your hands across your lower abdomen (the Tan Tien – see p. 42), men with the left hand on top, women with the right hand on top. You can slip the thumb of your top hand gently inside the palm of your other hand.

Alternatively you can stand with your weight on one leg, resting your hands lightly on your thighs so that two or three fingers are touching your leg. Bend your elbows very slightly away from your body. Always make a small "L" or "V" with your feet, so that there is an angle of 45 to 90 degrees between them.

STANDING UP

Support your weight by holding an overhead strap, a pole, a handle, or even by resting part of your body, such as your hips, against some part of the bus or train. Let as much as possible of your weight rest at that point. If you have a free hand, rest it inside your pocket or lightly against your thigh. Relax your entire body, allowing your weight to rest on the point that supports you, but not so that your grip or body becomes tense. Let your energy support you.

SITTING

Make sure you sit facing the direction in which the vehicle is moving.

Try to sit comfortably straight. Drop your shoulders. Rest your forearms on the armrests if you can, letting your palms drop down to hold an invisible balloon on your lap. Or let your wrists rest on your thighs, your palms turned slightly upward as if holding the underside of an invisible balloon between them. Relax and breathe naturally. Keep your eyes open and your mind alert.

Driving

YOUR HANDS ON THE WHEEL

Don't grip the wheel. Don't use strong muscle power to turn it. Let your fingers curve lightly around the wheel. Drop your shoulders and elbows. Let the tension in your upper arms, forearms, and wrists run off like water.

WAITING

This is an excellent moment to practise Zhan Zhuang. Whether both your hands are on the wheel or one is on the gear stick, adjust your palms and fingers to resemble an open, relaxed Zhan Zhuang position. For example, you can rest both arms and pretend you are holding a large balloon. If you tend to be very tense, try playing smooth-flowing music in your car. Keep your mind alert, your head floating lightly from the crown of your skull, and breathe calmly. Even a few moments will help your whole system.

Walking

If you want to refresh yourself, go for a walk and try the following. Slip the four fingers of each hand in your trouser pockets, leaving your thumbs outside. Rest the weight of your arms against the fabric of the pockets, keeping your elbows slightly away from the sides of your body. Walk slightly more slowly than usual. If possible, put your arms in one of the Zhan Zhuang positions and walk, holding your arms steady. If you can't find a convenient place to walk, stand in one position, hold the invisible balloon, and slowly mark time on the spot for two or three minutes.

On a bicycle

An upright bicycle is best for this exercise. As you ride, drop your weight into your lower body. Let your upper body rest, completely relaxed. Hold the handlebars with your thumbs and forefingers only (see below). Let your other fingers rest lightly over the bars, as if you were resting your palms and fingers on a floating balloon. Don't grip the handlebars unless you need to brake. Do all the work with your lower body. Imagine you are moving forward like a waterfowl on a pond: underneath you are circling your feet like a powerful paddle; above, your entire upper body is travelling effortlessly forward.

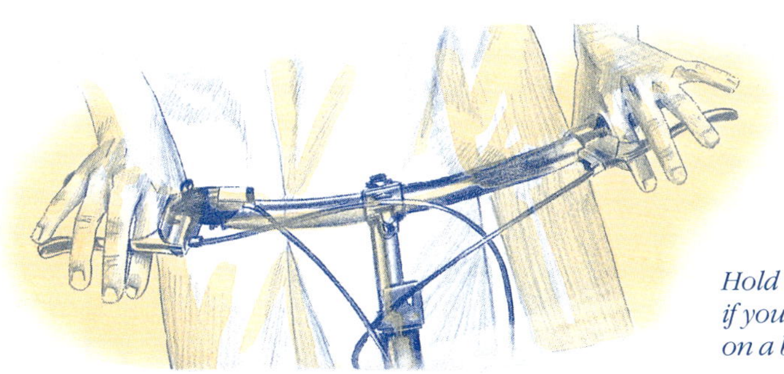

Hold the handlebars gently as if you were resting your palms on a balloon.

Leisure

You will derive enormous benefits from your Zhan Zhuang training in all your leisure activities: at home; in the garden; during and after sports; or when working on do-it-yourself projects. Applying Zhan Zhuang principles to your activities helps build stamina and alertness for sports; allows you to work more smoothly and safely on DIY jobs, for longer periods; and prevents backache after lifting and digging in the garden.

READING OR WATCHING TELEVISION

You can even practise Zhan Zhuang in an armchair. Sit straight, even if you rest against the back of the chair. Open your hands and let them hold the balloon gently in front of you. If there are no armrests, let your wrists lie on your thighs and hold the balloon in your lap. When you read, hold the book in your hands in front of you, always making sure that your arms and elbows are away from your body.

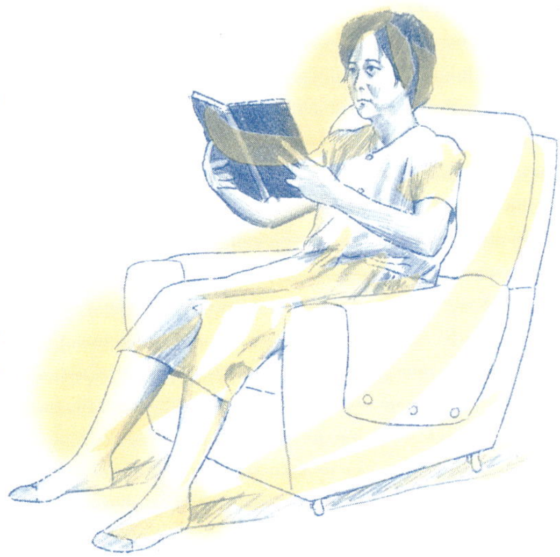

Hold your arms and elbows away from your body when you read.

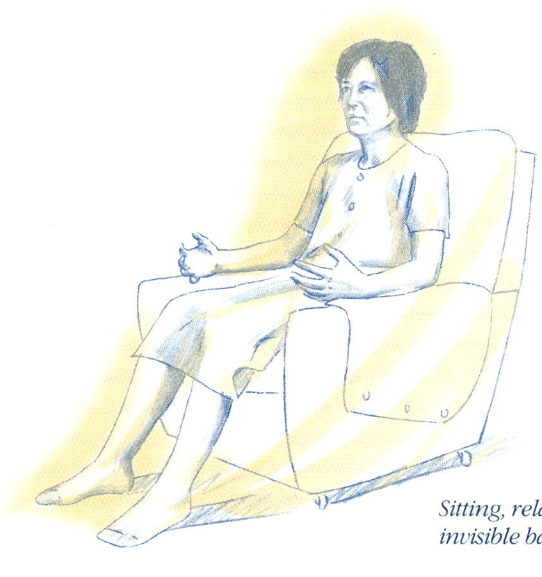

Sitting, relaxed, holding an invisible balloon.

Doing it yourself

Most DIY enthusiasts use a tremendous amount of muscle when they are gripping, hammering, and sawing – even when using electric tools. But you can usually work more smoothly, more safely, and for longer periods, if you apply the Way of Energy.

Take using a hammer, for instance. Most people simply grip the hammer as hard as they can and use every ounce of muscle to deliver the blow, constantly tensing their arm, wrist, and finger muscles. After a while their muscles begin to feel the pain and need a rest. The only comfort is the thought that all those aching muscles are slowly "turning to steel".

There is another way. The Way of Energy is the way of bamboo, not the way of steel. The bamboo is one of the strongest and most durable woods on our planet. It rarely breaks, yet it can bear enormous weights and survive fierce tropical typhoons. Instead of thinking of your hands and arms as pieces of steel, treat them like bamboo.

The principle outlined below – using maximum energy and minimum muscle – can be applied to dozens of other DIY and household tasks.

THE WAY OF BAMBOO
Hold the hammer only as firmly as necessary. Keep your wrist flexible. Think of your elbow and shoulder moving in small, flowing circles. Keep your eye on the target and then allow all the energy in your system to flow like a current down through your arm. Your joints and bones trace a pattern like a whip and the full force is transmitted in a single snap to the point of contact at the head of the hammer. The result is a deadly accurate blow, like the powerful slap of an unbreakable bamboo cane.

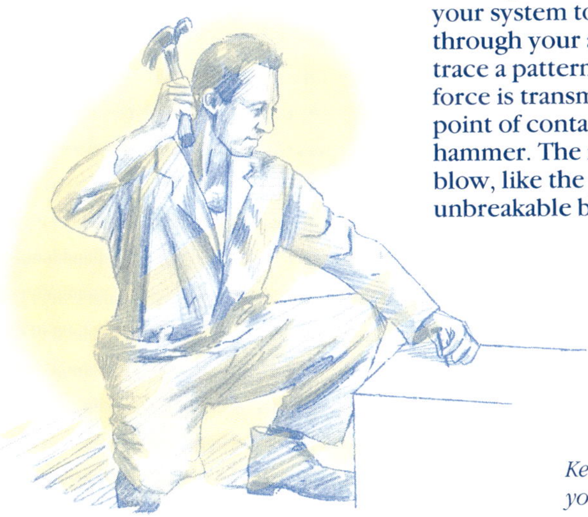

Keep your body supple, and your movements smooth.

Energy for sports

Because Zhan Zhuang training raises the level of energy in your body and greatly increases both your physical fitness and your mental alertness, it is an excellent fundamental training for anyone who plays sports or takes part in athletics of any sort.

If you are interested in building up your stamina and developing your capacity for vigorous individual or team sports, there are some aspects of Zhan Zhuang training that can be of particular value to you.

You can apply the principles and get the value of the exercise that follows when you are on the sports field, on the tennis court, or in the swimming pool.

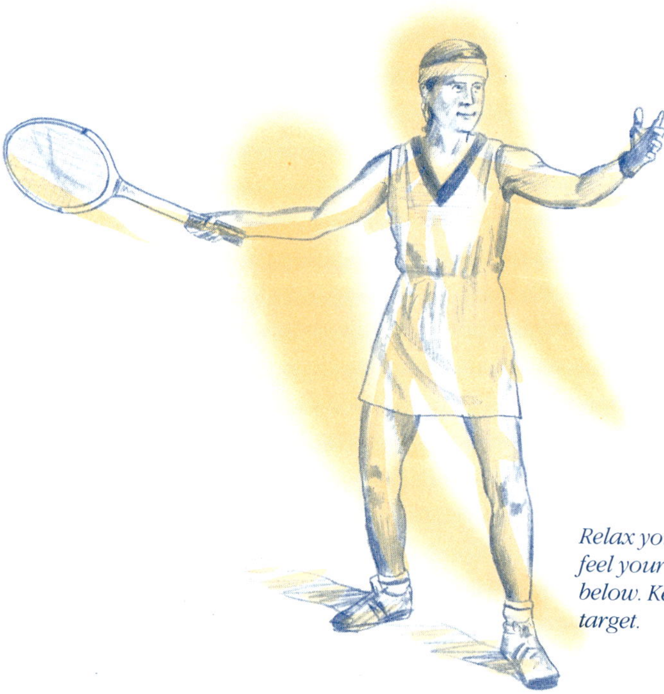

Relax your upper body and feel your strength come from below. Keep your eyes on the target.

SPORTS ROUTINE

Once you have learned the first two positions and are ready to start Ba Duan Jin (Chapter 4), try to do the Ba Duan Jin exercises every day. Follow this by a minimum of 20 minutes of the standing exercises. Begin with five minutes of the second position – Holding the Balloon (see pp. 34-35). Then work up to 15 minutes in the fifth position – Holding the Balloon in Front of your Face (see pp. 92-93). Sink down as low as you can. At first you may feel a little stiff and will not be able to sink very low. Don't worry, and don't force the position. Just sink down, taking care not to let your knees extend beyond your toes.

After a few minutes, you will find that you can sink lower. Your weight will naturally shift backward toward your heels. Once you have reached a lower position, hold it: do not rise up. If you feel pain or trembling in your legs, relieve it by sinking just a little lower.

Now bring your mind into the exercise. First, check that your hands, forearms, upper arms, shoulders, neck, and back are relaxed. This is easy to say, but very difficult to achieve. Concentrate your mind on telling each set of muscles to relax. This is vital training for all strenuous sports. Your upper body must remain weightless and relaxed, regardless of the strain you are under.

Second, without moving, tense every muscle in your legs so that they are as firm as rocks; feel maximum pressure in your thighs and your calves and grip the floor firmly with your toes. Grip and tense for five seconds, then relax. Grip and tense again for five seconds, then relax. Check that your upper body is utterly calm and unmoving. Continue working on your lower limbs until you have tensed and relaxed 30 times. This exercise is marvellous for strengthening the flow of energy in your legs and feet, building the power of your working muscles, and redirecting your centre of gravity downward to its original focus.

PRACTICAL TIPS

- Don't hunch your shoulders.

- Let your entire upper body be empty.

- If you are running, fix your eyes on the target and put your mind in your feet. Let your body disappear entirely.

- If you are swimming, keep your upper body loose. Keep your mind wholly on your "engine" – your legs and feet.

- If you are playing raquet sports, such as tennis or squash, keep your weight low. Relax your entire upper body, so there is no tension whatsoever in any of the vital joints such as your shoulders, neck, elbows, and wrists. Forget your hand: let all action flow effortlessly from below. That is the source of explosive power. Keep your eyes on your target, ignore the rest of your body, and let your feet be the only other points in your mind.

In the garden

People often experience back pain and tension in their arms and shoulders after working in the garden. You can help prevent this by doing the exercise described below.

If there are trees and bushes in or near your garden, their Chi, especially in the early morning, will be wonderful. They make an ideal place to do your Zhan Zhuang training.

BEFORE YOU BEGIN

Before you start gardening, stand still in the Wu Chi position for a minute (see p. 29). Then do the eighth Ba Duan Jin exercise (see p. 80): place the backs of your hands in the small of your back just above your hip bones, then bounce up and down from your knees so that you shake your whole torso – back and front – like jelly. Breathe out in short bursts through your nose. Keep shaking over 10 or 12 complete exhalations.

When gardening, try to keep your upper body relaxed. Use the power from your lower body to do the work. If you feel pain and stiffness in your back, stop. Take a break and do the shaking exercise.

Lifting heavy weights

At home, at your work place, or in your leisure activities, you are likely to have to lift a heavy weight at some point. It might be a box of papers or soft drinks; it might be a table or a piece of equipment. Whatever it is and whatever the circumstances, you can apply your knowledge of Zhan Zhuang to lift the weight more easily and help prevent injury.

POINTS TO REMEMBER

There are eight points to remember for both lifting and putting down heavy weights. Notice the difference in the sequence of breathing between lifting and lowering.

LIFTING

1. Relax your arms, shoulders, and upper body.

2. Let your weight sink into your lower body.

3. Squat down to grasp the object, keeping your back straight and relaxed.

4. Hold the object in against your body so it is in physical contact with you.

5. Breathe out before standing up.

6. Breathe in as you stand up, carrying the object up with you.

7. Stay still for a second after standing up. This is very important.

8. Before you move, be clear in your mind about the direction of your movement, then move. Your mind should move first.

COMPLETE THE MOVEMENT

It is essential to breathe in as you lift and to complete the lift fully before making any other movement. A lot of back injuries are caused by people moving sideways or at an angle while they are still lifting, or by merging the end of the upward movement with the beginning of the next movement. This can place great strain on the spine and cause dislocation. Be sure to complete the lift fully, and allow your mind to settle, before going on to your next movement.

LOWERING HEAVY WEIGHTS

1. Relax your arms, shoulders, and upper body.

2. Let your weight sink into your lower body.

3. Hold the object in contact with your body.

4. Breathe in, without moving.

5. Hold your breath as you squat down to lower the object.

6. When you have lowered the object to its new resting place, breathe out.

7. Pause for a second.

8. Breathe in as you stand up.

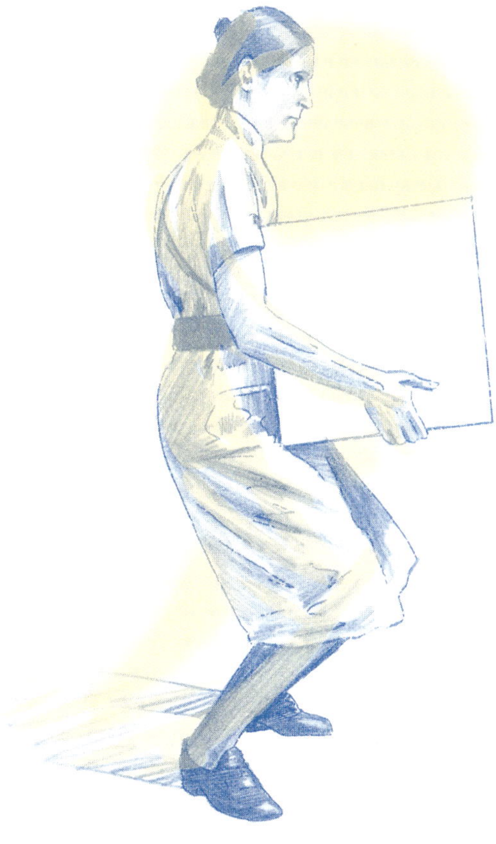

Hold the object in contact with your body, whether lifting or putting down a heavy object.

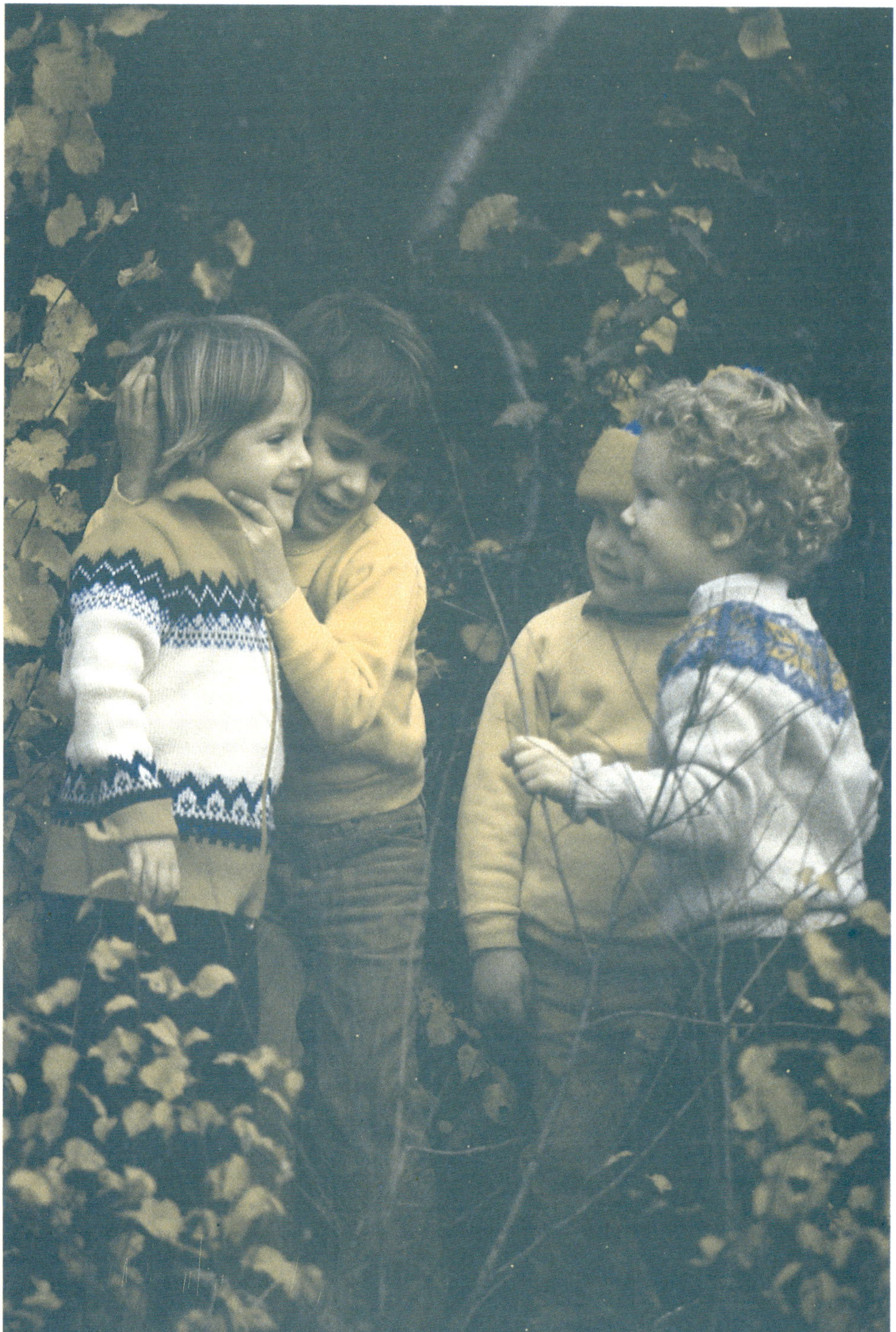

CHAPTER 9
THE LIFE CYCLE

We are surrounded by the cycles of nature. The transformation of day into night. The passage of the seasons. The promise of birth and the certainty of death. We, too, are points in the pattern of the cycle. Each of us – and every other living creature – is a prodigious enterprise of energy; flowing, adapting, and expressing itself through countless transmutations.

Our bodies are patterns of change – the ebb and flow of our breathing, the constant stream of messages sent and received by our nervous systems, the ceaseless renewal of our tissues, and the complex cycle of digestion. We are continually transforming and being transformed.

Nature constantly seeks to maintain a balance during these changes. In our bodies, this process is known (in Western science) as homeostasis. We are always adapting to subtle changes in the atmosphere and our environment, and also compensating for adjustments made elsewhere in our bodies.

The regular practice of Zhan Zhuang gives powerful support to this process. It helps all our vital systems to cope with the impact of a stressful, polluted, and debilitating daily environment. Whether you are an office worker, manager, manual labourer, homemaker, or performer, the long-term benefits of regular training will be unmistakable. If your internal organs are functioning harmoniously, your health will benefit and you will have high tolerance for stress. If you are relaxed under pressure, you will be more productive. And regular Zhan Zhuang practice will ensure that your power will be directed by a mind that is increasingly alert and sensitive.

The great cycle of our lives, from infancy to old age, affects all aspects of our energy – its vitality, the way it flows, and how we give form to it. Each of the parts of this cycle brings its own opportunities for taking up Zhan Zhuang: they are described in this chapter, along with guidelines and suggestions for how Zhan Zhuang can help you at all stages in your life.

Infants and children

Children are just bursting with energy. Sometimes they seem to have too much and simply don't know what to do with it. Often they have trouble getting some balance in their behaviour. It's easy for them to get carried away with extremes of frantic activity followed by sudden exhaustion, or to be injured falling down or running around. Doing a little Zhan Zhuang can make a big difference at this early age and greatly help the development of young children when their whole bodies are going through the stressful surges of rapid growth.

NO NEED TO WARM UP
There is no need for a young child to do the warm up exercises. Standing, Holding the Balloon, is enough. Don't worry, either, about getting all the little details of the posture correct. These are not necessary at this age. And it's not likely that a young child will have the time, patience, or disposition to do any Zhan Zhuang in the mornings. At bedtime, however, some Zhan Zhuang may be possible and will prove to be beneficial.

PARENTS AND CHILDREN
Try some of the standing exercises with your child or children. The effect on them is likely to be pacifying and help them to sleep. Try reading them a story while they stand. Their minds will be on the story, and you will find that they can stand right through it. They'll probably be calm and ready to sleep. The chances are they will have good dreams as well.

An added benefit of the whole family standing together, even briefly, in the early evening is that it prepares the children for sleep, but at the same time helps to recharge the parents' energy for the rest of the evening!

ACCIDENTS
If your child has a minor accident, such as a tumble, ask him or her to stand in one of the Zhan Zhuang positions for a few moments. This will help the circulation, reduce bruising, and help restore some self-control, regardless of the initial shock and tears.

POOR POSTURE
Sleeping on a hard bed at an early age stretches the spine and so helps to prevent poor posture. It pays off handsomely in later years. Regular Zhan Zhuang exercise will help correct poor posture later, but you can avoid this sort of problem by cultivating good alignment when young.

Children benefit from Zhan Zhuang exercise, especially before going to bed.

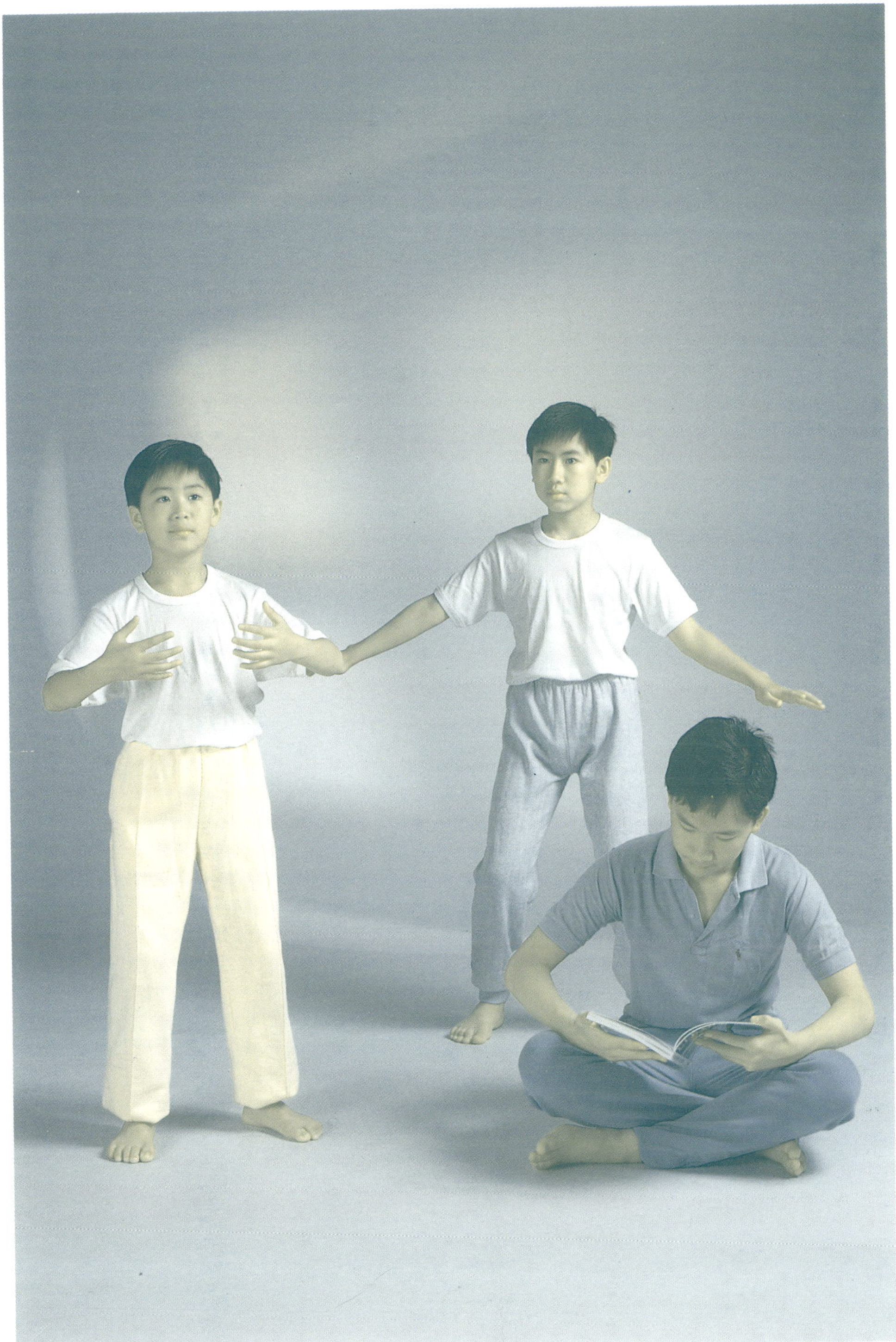

Teenagers

A young person going through the teen years is under great mental and physical stress. It is a time of rapid growth, much of it decisive for the long-term welfare of the person in later life. There are sexual and other hormonal changes. The bone structure reaches its final stage of expansive growth. It is common for teenagers to grow in spurts – a period of fast growth for several weeks may be followed by several days of illness or sheer exhaustion. Both their mental and emotional life, too, may undergo profound changes. And social pressures on the individual change considerably: new opportunities and dangers are suddenly present.

RESTORING BALANCE

Zhan Zhuang training can be extremely useful in regulating and smoothing the entire growth process in the teenage period. It helps to calm the nervous system and restore balance in the body's energy network. Because it strengthens the body's immune system, regular Zhan Zhuang training will be a great asset in this period when the body can easily find itself vulnerable to stress-related ailments or diseases such as asthma and headaches.

CONTROLLING TEMPER

A further useful effect of practising Zhan Zhuang is the help it can give people in controlling their temper. In these difficult teenage years, a young person's emotional balance may be easily disturbed. Sudden rages are common, as are other bouts of strong emotion that seem wildly out of all proportion. The powerful effect of Zhan Zhuang keeps the disposition more steady and helps young people to cope with the world around them with less pain.

ENERGY FOR SPORTS

Zhan Zhuang at this stage of life has the additional advantage of giving strong foundations for all sporting and athletic activities (see p. 154). It boosts the internal energy. And, in my experience, it usually has the natural effect of stopping young people smoking.

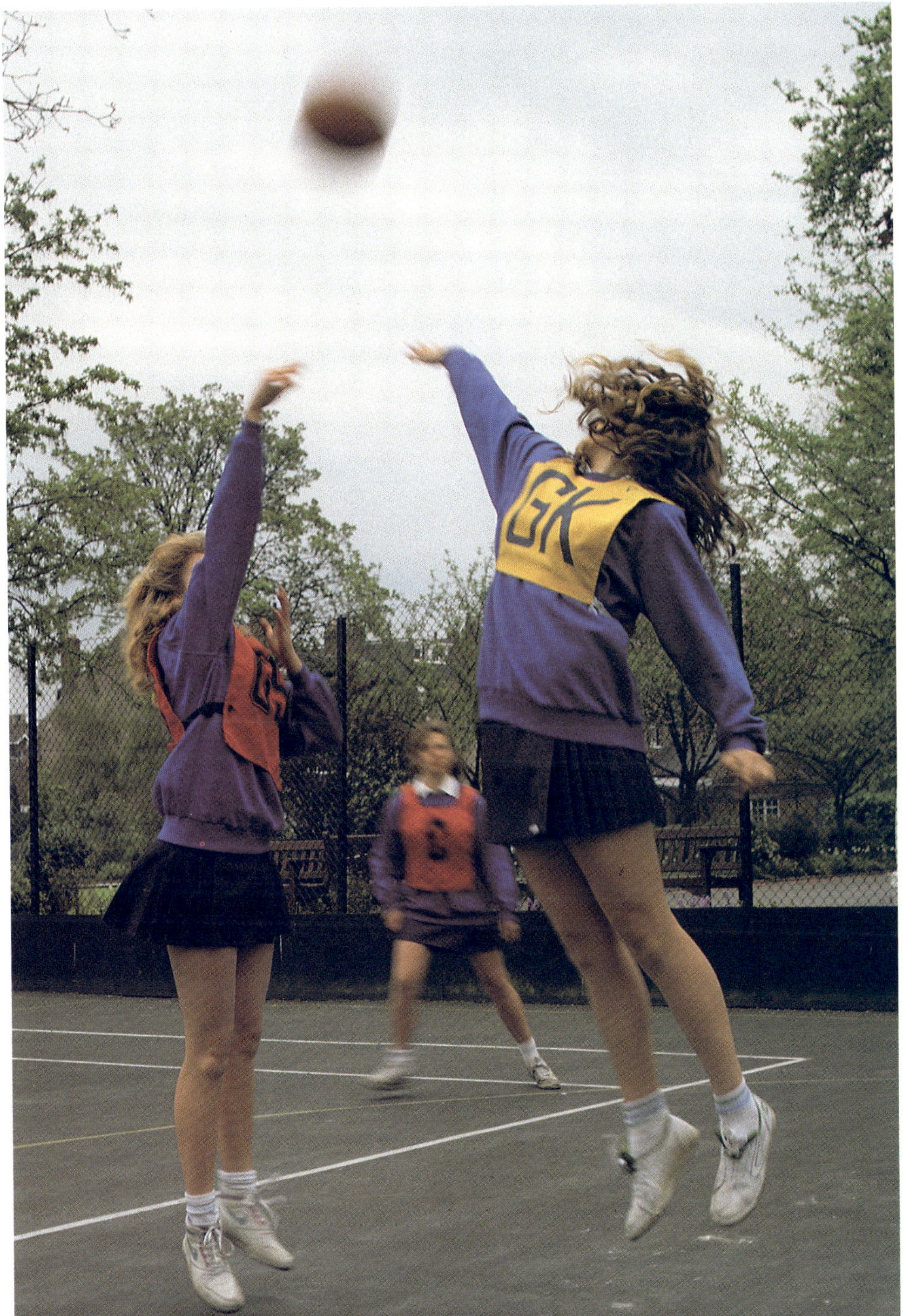
GK

Zhan Zhuang for women

Unlike some exercise systems, which treat women and men differently, Zhan Zhuang can be practised in exactly the same way by both sexes. Because of a woman's child-bearing capacity, there are some special circumstances in her life where Zhan Zhuang exercises can be of particular help – before and during menstrual periods and in connection with childbirth.

THE MENSTRUAL CYCLE

The menstrual cycle causes major changes in a woman's body every month. Many women experience pain during their periods, and tension beforehand, and suffer from irregularity of the whole cycle. The practice of both Ba Duan Jin and Zhan Zhuang exercises has been shown to make a marked improvement in the cycle. Periods become much more regular. The pain is eased. The pre-menstrual days are far less tense and difficult. The whole flow of energy in the woman's body is strengthened and regulated as it adjusts to the hormonal and internal physical changes at these points in the month.

BA DUAN JIN

If you experience a lot of period pain, try the following three exercises when the pain occurs. Begin with the first Ba Duan Jin exercise: Supporting the Sky with Both Hands Regulates all Internal Organs. This is described on pages 66 to 67. Then, do the second Ba Duan Jin exercise: Drawing a Bow to Each Side. This is explained on pages 68 to 69. Finish with the eighth Ba Duan Jin exercise: Shaking the Body Wards Off all Illnesses, described on page 80. The effect of these three exercises is to adjust the position of all the internal organs and to release accumulated tension.

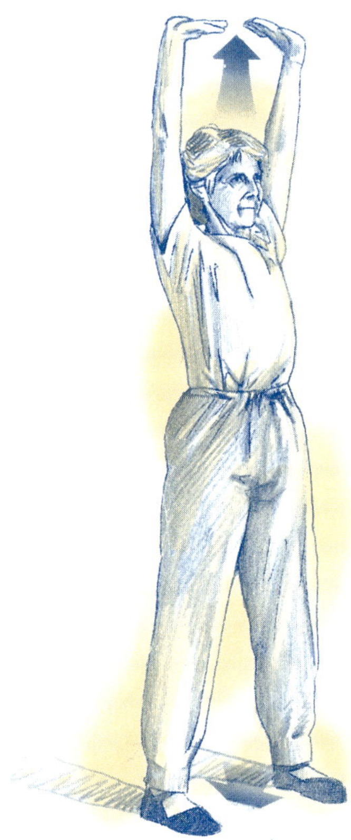

1. The first Ba Duan Jin exercise, Supporting the Sky with Both Hands Regulates all Internal Organs, will help ease period pains.

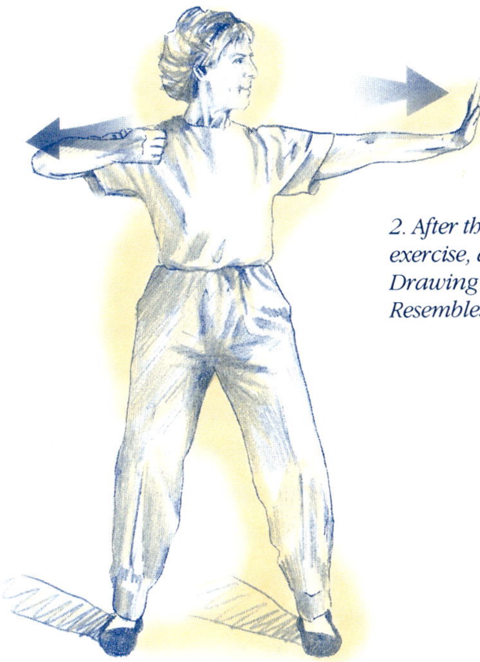

2. After the first Ba Duan Jin exercise, do the second: Drawing a Bow to Each Side Resembles Shooting an Eagle.

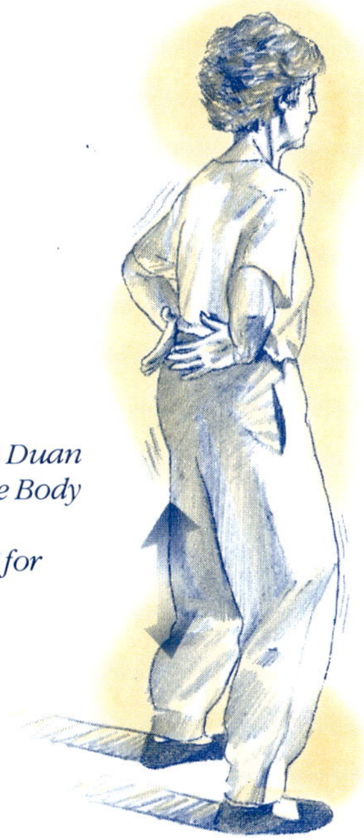

3. Finally, the eighth Ba Duan Jin exercise, Shaking the Body Wards Off all Illnesses, completes the sequence for easing the pains.

Pregnancy

When you are pregnant a selective combination of Ba Duan Jin and Zhan Zhuang exercises practised every day will be a great help to you and to your baby.

PREPARING FOR CHILDBIRTH

This combination of exercises is excellent for preparing mother and child for birth. It helps to build energy for labour and, by helping anchor the centre of energy in the body, it develops strength in your lower body.

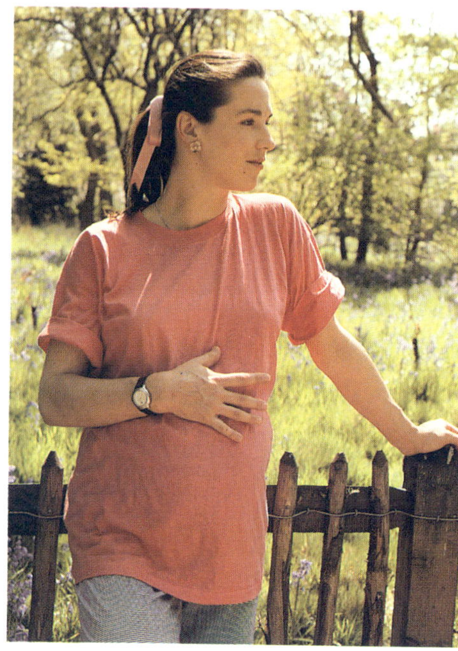

Begin with these three Ba Duan Jin exercises.
CAUTION: Do not practise the other Ba Duan Jin exercises after learning that you are pregnant.

1. Supporting the Sky with Both Hands Regulates all Internal Organs (see pp. 66-67)
2. Drawing a Bow to Each Side Resembles Shooting an Eagle (see pp. 68-69)
3. Holding Up a Single Hand Regulates the Spleen and Stomach (see pp. 70-71)

Follow these with up to 20 minutes of standing in either:

the second position – Holding the Balloon (see pp. 34-35)
the third position – Holding Your Belly (see pp. 84-85)
or
the fourth position – Standing in the Stream (see pp. 88-89)

After childbirth

Having given birth, your whole system goes through enormous changes. You have given a great deal of your energy to your baby, so it is essential to build up your own vitality again.

RECOVERING YOUR ENERGY

As soon as you feel able, try doing some Zhan Zhuang while sitting or lying down. Just hold the imaginary balloon for as long as you feel comfortable. Then, one month after giving birth, and as long as your recovery is progressing normally, begin doing the full sequence of Ba Duan Jin and Zhan Zhuang exercises. This combination will be of immense help in regulating your internal energy, helping you to adjust to the next stage of your life, and restoring your vital force.

Practise the second position – Holding the Balloon, while lying down if this is most comfortable for you.

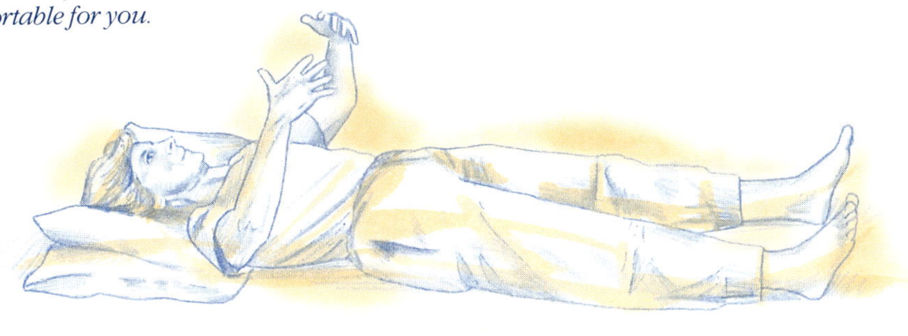

Lie with your knees up (see below) or flat on the ground (see above). If you raise your knees, bring your toes off the ground as well.

If this is too difficult, rest your elbows and the soles of your feet on the bed, keeping your knees bent.

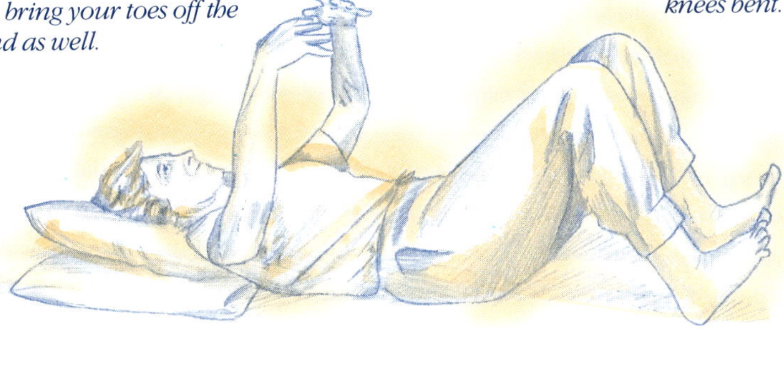

Your middle age

The years around fifty can be crucial in a person's life. A surprising number of people reach this age and suddenly experience a kind of rapid deterioration and collapse. Some who have had a very hard early life are victims of sudden death through heart attacks and other violent traumas. Many more experience a range of other problems such as spinal pain, frozen shoulders, high blood pressure, loss of self-control, chronic illness, severe depression, and lassitude. All the pressures of life seem to converge at this point in a person's existence.

This vital juncture can also be the start of a second life. An ideal time to consider starting Zhan Zhuang training is, therefore, in your forties or very early fifties. The result at this period in life can be profound.

People who have practised Zhan Zhuang or other forms of Chi Kung seem to change from within and instead of getting older they seem to start getting younger. Their faces become brighter and smoother. Their sexual energy revives. Chi Kung masters, at the age of 70 or 80, often look far, far younger than their years. They reveal great energy when they walk. Their temperament is calm and some are able to work harder and longer than adults twenty years younger than themselves!

THE BEGINNINGS

So what exactly do you do if you want to try Zhan Zhuang at this stage of your life? First of all, don't confuse it with aerobic and muscle-building exercises – neither the effect nor the experience is the same. Don't expect that sort of sweat and pain. The second thing to bear in mind is that Zhan Zhuang works at a very deep level, tackling profound inner disorders. So if you have accumulated the effects of 40 or 50 years of stress, bad posture, illnesses, and all the other headaches of daily life, you can expect a lot of unusual sensations once you start your training. These are described in Chapter 3. Your entire body, mind, and nervous system are in for a complete overhaul.

The single most difficult thing to get over is your own mental resistance. You are changing the energy habits of a lifetime. Over the first few months you will go through a whole range of thoughts and feelings, many rebelling against your decision to stand still! Don't give in; remember that rising to a new level of mental stamina is also part of this system of mind body exercise.

WEEKLY PLAN

You can help yourself by making a weekly plan. Start at Chapter 1 and work out how long you will spend daily on the two warm up exercises and then the Wu Chi, or first position (see pp. 28-29). For example, you might spend six or seven minutes on the gentle warm ups and five minutes standing in the Wu Chi position. Just do that each day for the first week as the first step in your journey.

Don't expect miraculous results at the end of your first week. Just having taken the first step – and stuck to it – will be a great achievement. Then review the advice in Chapter 1 and make a plan for your next week's training.

If you follow this idea, you will find that you can set your own natural pace and make authentic, careful progress through the exercises in this book. The results are subtle but unmistakable. It is usually said that after 100 days of Chi Kung exercise most people can be sure to see results.

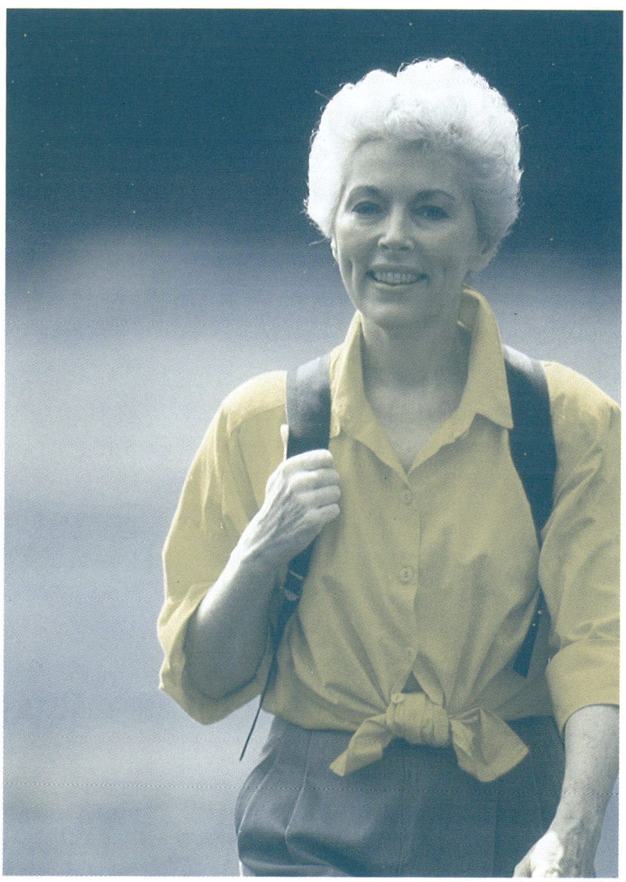

A ripe old age

As we age we usually begin to suffer all sorts of ailments. Difficulty with walking is common, as are digestion troubles, high blood pressure, brittle bones, incontinence, and low energy.

Even if you take up Zhan Zhuang at an advanced age, you will feel the benefits. Your digestion will improve, as will your bladder control, and your bones will strengthen. You are almost certain to feel that your energy is being restored, that you feel younger in yourself, and that you have an increasing measure of self-control. Many older people also report great improvement in their sleeping patterns.

STARTING TO PRACTISE

What is the best way for an elderly person to start practising Zhan Zhuang? You should devote yourself to the warm up exercises and the first five positions described in this book. Practise for a maximum of only 5 to 10 minutes at a time. Just as you are advised to change your eating habits so that you have smaller meals more frequently, so with Zhan Zhuang – you should try standing for 5 to 10 minutes several times in the course of the day.

Depending on your age and level of fitness, you may need to experiment with the sitting or lying positions (see pp. 142 and 167) at first and then move on to standing at a later stage.

COMMON PROBLEMS

You may feel pain in your shoulders or knees. Don't be put off by this. It is perfectly natural. If the pain is too great, gently bring your standing session to an end by standing in the Wu Chi position.

Sometimes your breathing can become forced or you may start to feel a little breathless. If this occurs, take it as a signal that you have reached a natural limit and gently bring your Zhan Zhuang session to a close in the Wu Chi position as before.

If you feel dizzy while standing, you should gently stop, walk slowly, and if necessary sit down. Don't close your eyes. This sensation can be caused by an unusually strong current of energy in your system. It is not necessarily something to be upset about.

If you feel the need for some support while standing, you can rest your bottom against the edge of a high stool or use the type of walking stick that opens out into a little seat. Holding the arm positions alone will stimulate your energy circulation.

RAPID IMPROVEMENT

A particularly widespread problem among older people is dry, itchy skin. Especially at night in bed, many older people suffer dreadfully from constant itching of the skin. It can last all night. Even if an older person with this problem has never done any form of Chi Kung, a brief period of regular Zhan Zhuang practice will ease the itching and may help to remove it altogether. One 86-year-old in China said that he had been scratching his skin every night for ten years, but that after only a few days of Zhan Zhuang exercise he had finally started sleeping through a whole night without scratching.

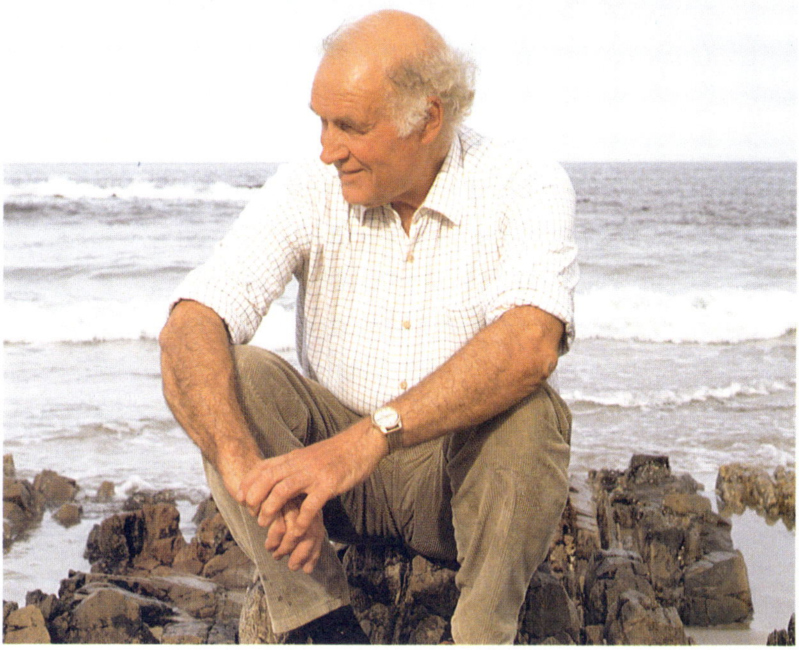

A WORD OF CAUTION

Positions 6 to 9 in this book have a strong effect on your circulatory system and, as with all intense exercise, push up your blood pressure during the period of training. Attempt these positions only if your doctor advises that your normal blood pressure level will permit this. This is not a problem for positions 1 to 5, the warm ups, or any of the "mentality exercises" (Chapter 2) – in fact, these will be positively beneficial for any problem in your cardiovascular system.

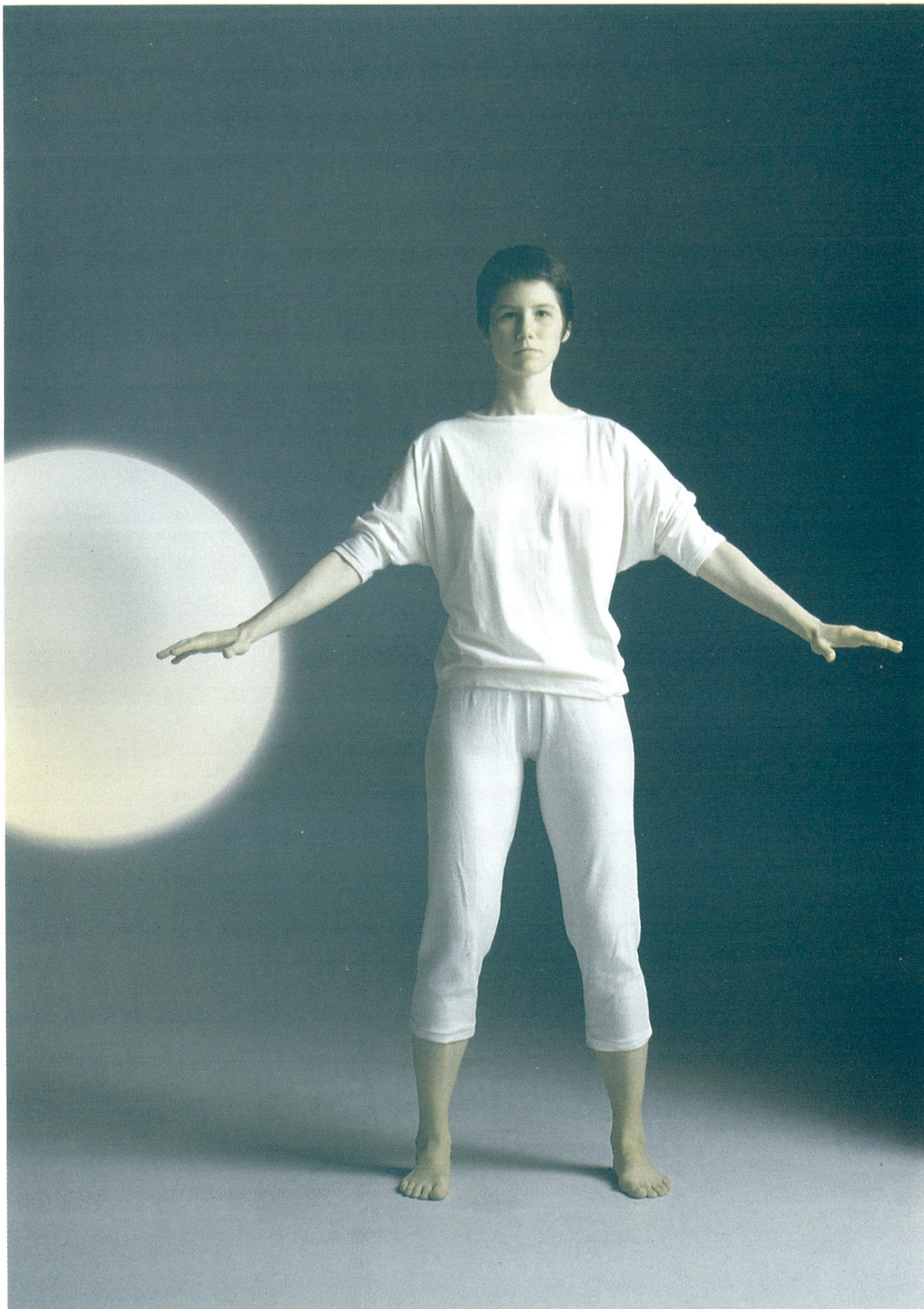

CHAPTER 10
TAKING CARE OF YOURSELF

There are a number of practical steps you can take in everyday life to help keep your energy system balanced and healthy. It is important to prevent disease, not merely to wait until you have an ailment and then try to cure it. The traditional approach of Chinese medicine was to pay the doctor to keep you healthy and if you became ill the payments would cease until you were well again! The fundamental reason for doing the exercises in this book is to strengthen your internal power, immunity, and stamina so that you live a life of health as long as possible.

Your whole body functions with an extraordinarily complex central heating system. Obviously we are not talking about a collection of pipes, tubes, and wires. Each of us is alive thanks to a beautifully organized biological system with its own delicate feedback mechanisms. These are reacting simultaneously to both internal changes and those in the environment.

Taking care of yourself begins with careful maintenance of your biological engine. The common-sense advice that follows at the beginning of this chapter pays attention to your eating and drinking (the fuel), to your temperature (the regulation of internal heating), and to tension (which can so easily cause blockages in internal circulation). Some of the bad habits we fall into by adulthood and which harm our biological engines can be eased by the practice of Zhan Zhuang. These are described later in the chapter, on page 175; others are included to highlight the range of influences that can damage your health.

The Ba Duan Jin exercises for self treatment that are outlined in the rest of the chapter will improve respiratory disorders, digestion problems, conditions of your circulatory and nervous systems, and some of the common problems connected with your bones and joints.

When convalescing, adapt your Zhan Zhuang exercises as shown on pages 186-187 to ease any difficulties in holding the normal positions. Useful first aid tips complete the chapter.

Maintaining your health

In addition to regular Zhan Zhuang practice, there are a number of straightforward steps you can take to keep your whole internal system in balance. These help to regulate the generation and flow of your energy.

KEEPING AN EVEN TEMPERATURE

Don't let yourself become extremely cold or hot. When you go out in winter and summer, protect yourself from sustained exposure to temperature extremes. In summer, if you are very hot and sweaty from exercise, keep your clothes on until you can cool down naturally, wash, and change. Don't strip off and let all your perspiration evaporate in the air. When you are hot and thirsty, don't take ice-cold drinks. They may be pleasant in your mouth, but they are a tremendous shock to your digestive system. As a general principle, it is best never to drink them. You should drink liquids at room temperature or, for relaxation, hot water or hot tea.

CONTROLLING TENSION

If you are doing a job that involves a lot of tension or concentration, be sure to take a break at least every two hours. Stop for five minutes and do the "energy wash" exercise described on page 145. It is essential to take such a break to allow your nervous system to calm down.

TIPS ON FOOD

In the morning, before breakfast, drink one or two glasses of pure or freshly filtered water at room temperature. The benefit of this to your system will be greatly enhanced by taking a spoonful of honey as well. Take it once a day, each morning before breakfast.

Never overeat. Never fill your stomach to its capacity at any one meal. Don't swallow your food rapidly; chew it thoroughly before swallowing. This makes it much easier for your stomach to digest. The Chinese way is to use aromatics (such as ginger, spring onions, and garlic) to help digestion, but not to use hot spices in cooking. Too many spices can cause digestive problems.

After eating, take a slow walk for a few minutes. Several small cups of hot Chinese tea (without milk) will also help to soothe your digestion.

RELAXATION BEFORE YOU SLEEP

Before sleeping, spend a minute or two massaging your abdomen. This brings many benefits to your digestive system and other internal organs. Place one hand over the other on your belly and make 36 anticlockwise circles and then 36 clockwise circles. You can do this standing, sitting, or lying down.

Bad habits

We grow up with so many pressures around us, that by the time we are adult many of us have lost touch with the functioning of our own bodies. We no longer know what is natural and what is not. The mass production, advertising, and sale of such a variety of food and other commodities, have created a new, fast-moving environment in which we are inundated with images, products, and services. People are constantly looking for ways to do things faster. A lifestyle based on this obsession has become so ingrained that it seems "natural". But there is a great difference between these ingrained habits and the way of nature.

Most of us develop techniques for "coping" with these and other stresses in our lives. Such techniques include smoking, alcohol, or sometimes even losing control of ourselves. We also ignore advice on food and diet. Some of our bad habits are described below, with reminders of how Zhan Zhuang can help.

Smoking This does lasting damage to the lungs and cardiovascular system, which are so vital to the circulation of Chi in your body that you should avoid undermining your health in this way. Many people who practise Zhan Zhuang regularly find that they lose their taste for tobacco and gradually drop the habit.

Narcotics Drugs do not contribute to a natural, healthy life. Most of them place a strain on your body and all of them affect the functioning of your central nervous system.

Alcohol and other depressants
Dependency on alcohol or other types of depressant can lead to extremely serious medical problems, as well as severely reducing the natural alertness of your mind. Dependency is a gradual process and therefore many people find that they have become addicts without having realized the route they were following.

Poor diet Many people pick up bad eating habits early in life. It is up to each individual to decide what is best, but one thing is certain: if you want a healthy life, you won't get it by eating rubbish!

Mind and emotions out of control
There is a tremendous difference between a rich inner life that results in the natural expression of emotion, and the kind of mental or emotional outburst that betrays serious internal disturbance. Such outbursts may seem a spontaneous, even necessary, release of feelings, but the person may in fact be a victim of behaviour patterns in which he or she is trapped. The regular practice of Zhan Zhuang will greatly aid the calm functioning of your nervous system, but it is wise to be alert to your mental and emotional habits. Your thoughts, moods, and emotions are part of your energy system and need to be in balance just as much as the rest of you!

Self-treatment

Many common ailments are signals that there is a temporary fault in your internal central-heating system. In the Chinese medical tradition, many complaints are dealt with by paying careful attention to the patterns of energy circulation through the system. Pain, for example, is treated as a signal of a blockage or stagnation at some point in the energy flow. Since Zhan Zhuang exercise is designed to enhance the flow of your energy and help regulate your internal balance, it can help deal with certain types of common ailments.

The pages that follow describe how to deal with problems in your respiratory system (below and opposite); your digestion (p. 178); your nervous system (pp. 180-182); your circulation (p. 183); and your bones and joints (p. 184).

Respiratory disorders

COMMON COLDS

As soon as you feel a cold coming you should avoid all milk products, since these stimulate mucus production. Then try the following regime in the evening. Drink one or two glasses of freshly filtered or purified water with a spoonful of honey. Have a long, hot bath. After drying off, put on a tracksuit, pyjamas, or other loose-fitting leisure wear. Stand in one of the Zhan Zhuang positions for as long as you can. Try to stand in that one position for a longer time than usual. For example, if you normally hold one of the standing positions for 20 minutes, listen to a half-hour tape or watch a 30-minute television programme while standing. Then go to sleep. Do your normal training next morning and repeat the anti-cold procedure in the evening, if necessary.

If you have a very bad cold, take your hot bath after standing in the Zhan Zhuang position. First stand as long as you possibly can, until you are sweating. Then dry off all the sweat and take a very hot bath (as hot as you can bear it), before going to sleep.

COUGHS

If you want to shake off a cough, try doing the following. First, do the second Ba Duan Jin exercise: Drawing a Bow to Each Side (see pp. 68-69). Keep your palms and fingers at right angles to your extended arms in order to get the maximum stretch in your wrists. After that, swing both your arms up slowly, then around in a full circle, 20 to 30 times. Finally, place both your hands, one on top of the other, over your throat. Slowly and firmly slide them down from your throat to the middle of your chest. Repeat this last action 8 to 10 times.

The effect of these simple exercises is first to build up your energy, then to use it to calm down the "rebellious Chi" rising up in your chest and throat.

ASTHMA

If you suffer from asthma, you should do the full set of eight Ba Duan Jin exercises every day. These are marvellous for your whole system and are well known for their long-term effect on anyone who suffers from chronic, debilitating conditions such as this.

In the short term, to help you with your present condition, you should first stand in the second Zhan Zhuang position – Holding the Balloon (see pp. 34-35), for two minutes. Then, do the first Ba Duan Jin exercise: Supporting the Sky with Both Hands (see pp. 66-67). Pay careful attention to the full stretch, which helps inhalation. Follow this with the third Ba Duan Jin exercise: Holding Up a Single Hand (see pp. 70-71). Again, pay careful attention to the full stretch required in the exercise. Finally, do the eighth exercise: Shaking the Body (see p. 80).

You must try to do these exercises every day in addition to regular Zhan Zhuang training. This is particularly important in view of the persistent, recurring nature of asthma. Over time, you will see the difference.

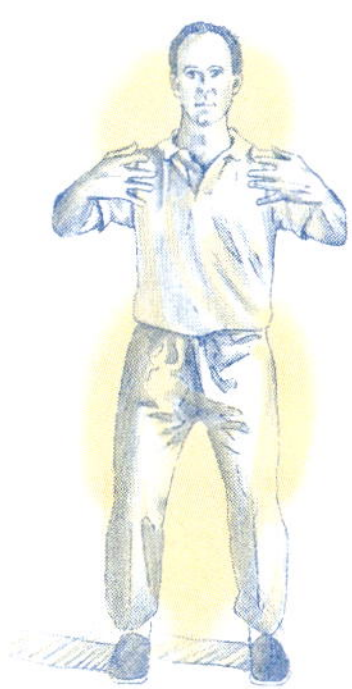

Holding the Balloon

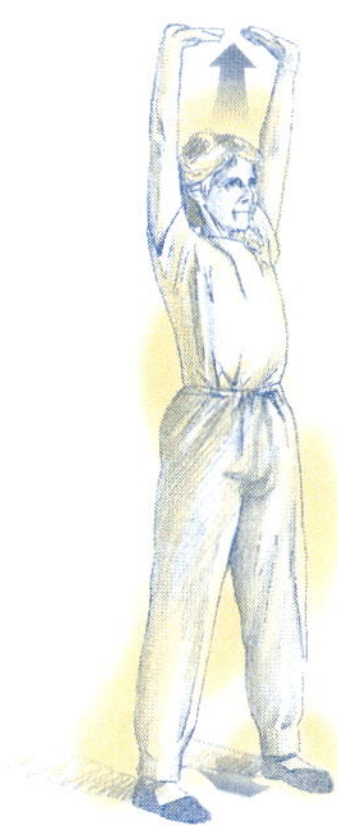

1st Ba Duan Jin

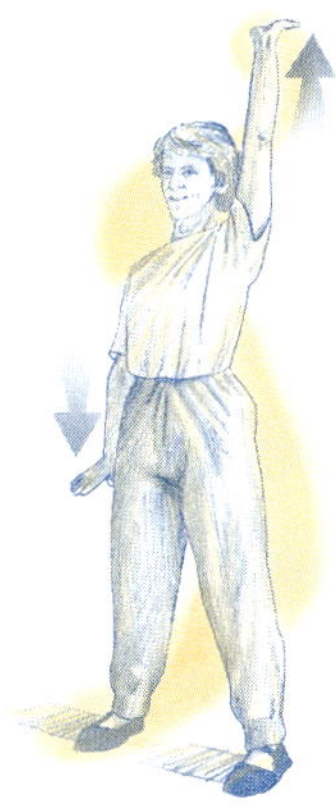

3rd Ba Duan Jin

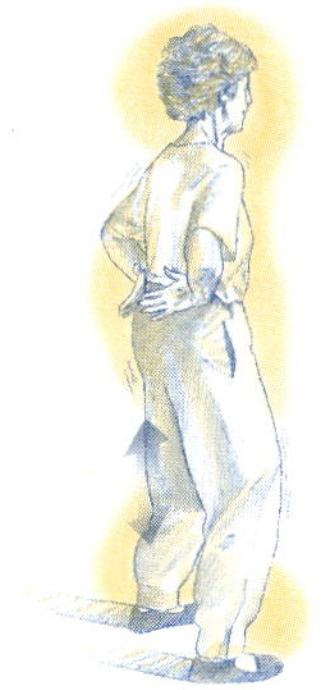

8th Ba Duan Jin

MEDICAL BENEFITS

Most people find that their breathing becomes deeper, slower, and more vigorous as a result of Zhan Zhuang training. Over time, like top athletes, their breathing rate reduces from 10 to 20 times per minute to 4 to 6 times. In one study the measurement of the volume of ventilation showed an increase of 33 per cent. Breathing becomes smoother as the movement of the diaphragm becomes more powerful (see also "Medical Benefits", p. 183).

Zhan Zhuang exercise is being used successfully in some hospitals in China for the treatment of tuberculosis and chronic ailments such as bronchial asthma.

Digestion

INDIGESTION AND NAUSEA

Indigestion and nausea are often caused by abdominal pressure. To relieve the symptoms, first stand for only two or three minutes in the second position – Holding the Balloon (see pp. 34-35). Then place both your hands, one on top of the other, on your belly just below your breastbone, and then rub your stomach as explained on page 174.

If you have a lot of stomach pain or think you are about to vomit, then squat down against the nearest wall (see below, right). Your feet should be flat on the ground and your lower back should rest against the wall. Let your forearms rest on top of your knees, or gently grasp your hands in front of your knees. Stay like that for a few minutes. It is a surprisingly restful position and has a powerful effect on abdominal discomfort.

Some people experience pain in the stomach if they are hungry, miss a regular meal, or have a long delay before eating. The pain will be eased by standing in the second Zhan Zhuang position for two minutes and then squatting against the wall for a few minutes.

Squatting with your lower back against a wall is surprisingly restful and will help abdominal discomfort.

WEIGHT PROBLEMS

Some people worry a great deal about their weight. For some this is just another form of anxiety. Others have real weight problems and need either to gain or lose weight. The regular practice of Zhan Zhuang naturally adjusts your body's metabolism and helps, over time, to bring you to your appropriate weight. The whole Zhan Zhuang system plus Ba Duan Jin will produce this effect – not overnight like a crash diet, but carefully and naturally as your entire body adjusts to its new state of health.

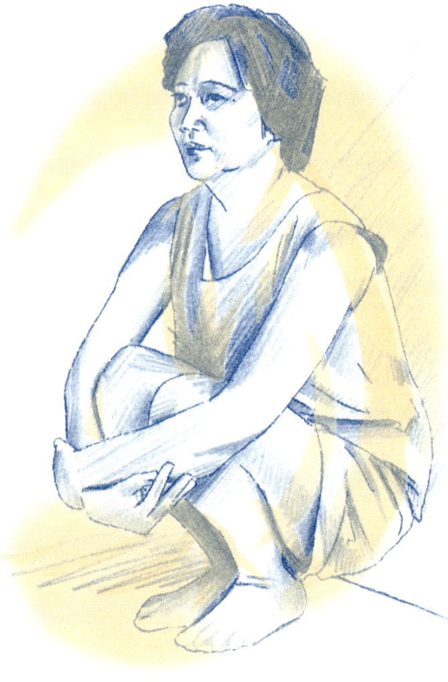

CONSTIPATION

Usually constipation results from inadequate movement in the digestive system. Try Zhan Zhuang to encourage proper internal movement. First stand either in the second position – Holding the Balloon (see pp. 34-35) or in the third position – Holding your Belly (see pp. 84-85). Stand still for two or three minutes. Relax your upper body. Then slowly tighten and relax the muscle of your rectum. Continue to do this as you stand. It should be the only muscle moving in your body. The movement will have a very strong effect on the rest of your intestinal tract.

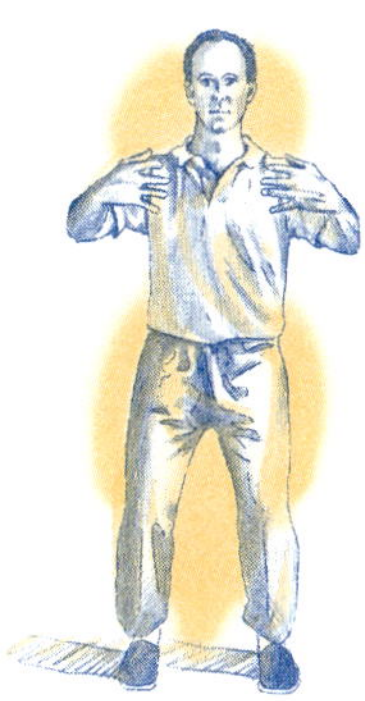

Holding the Balloon

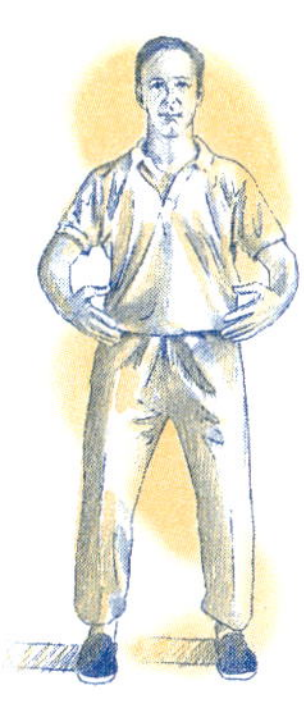

Holding your Belly

MEDICAL BENEFITS

Students of Zhan Zhuang usually notice increased digestive activity. This results from the strengthening and balancing of the contractions that pass food through the intestines. The major benefit is to reduce the likelihood of diseases of the gastro-intestinal tract and to regulate daily digestion. Medical studies in China have shown that Zhan Zhuang exercise is excellent for the relief of constipation. Patients who had bowel movements only once every three days or even less frequently, resumed a daily movement after starting basic exercises. Zhan Zhuang is also used in the treatment of gastric and duodenal ulcers.

NERVOUS SYSTEM

HEADACHES

If you have a headache there is a sequence of four practical steps you can take to ease the pain and eventually clear it completely. In my experience, following these steps helps relieve the symptoms of headaches, even migraines, in eight out of ten cases.

First, stand in the second Zhan Zhuang position – Holding the Balloon (see pp. 34-35), for two minutes. This is essential to build up your blood and, therefore, Chi circulation.

Second, do the fourth Ba Duan Jin exercise: Looking Back Like a Cow Gazing at the Moon. Follow the directions given on pages 72 to 73. This exercise helps to stimulate your central nervous system and to clear any blockages that may be affecting your spinal column and neck.

Third, do the eighth Ba Duan Jin exercise: Shaking the Body Wards Off all Illnesses (see p. 80). This is ideal for massaging your whole back, aiding your circulation, and helping you to relax from the top of your head down through your trunk.

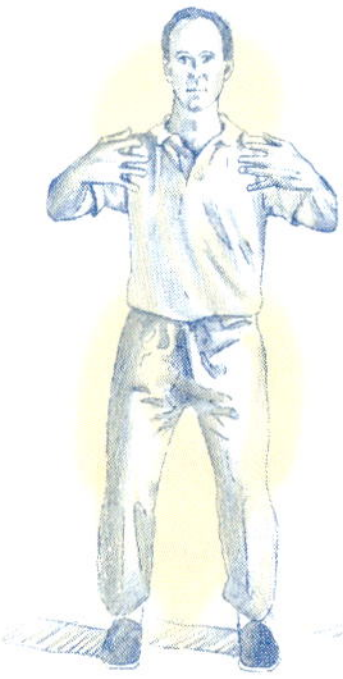

Holding the Balloon

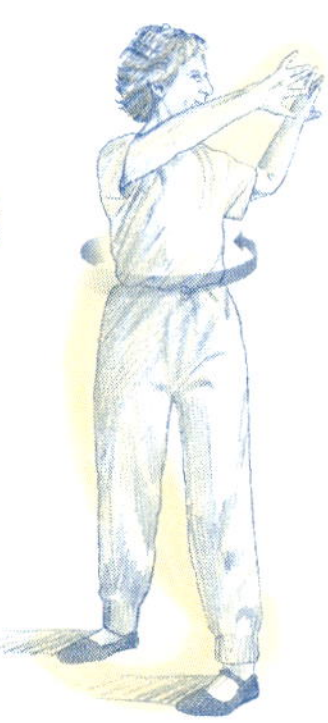

4th Ba Duan Jin

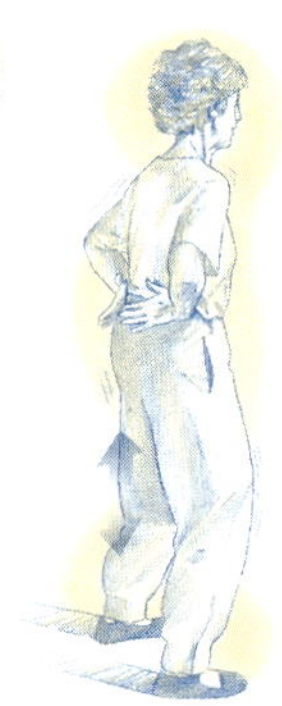

8th Ba Duan Jin

Fourth, place your open palms over your temples. Press them lightly against your head and gently massage the area around your temples. You will feel the effect of your Chi and are likely to notice a considerable improvement in your headache.

For most people, the pain will go completely after following these steps.

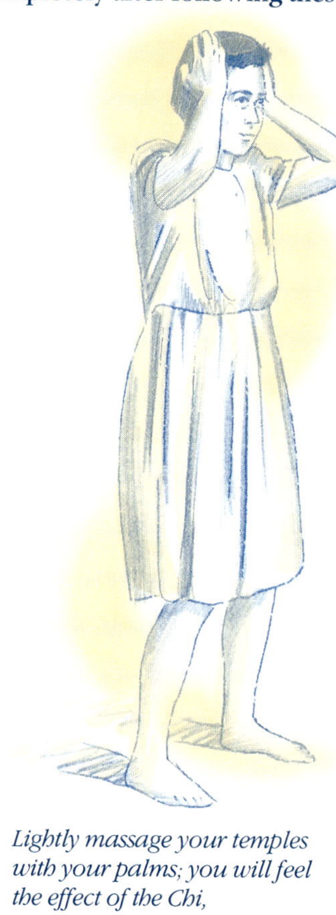

Lightly massage your temples with your palms; you will feel the effect of the Chi, heightened by the first three exercises.

HANGOVERS

It's the morning after. Your head is unbearable. You feel dizzy. You feel dehydrated and sick.

First, pour yourself a large glass of freshly-filtered or purified water (not refrigerated). Add a spoonful of honey. Drink it slowly.

Second, slowly swing your arms up and then back round in large circles 30 to 50 times.

Third, stand in the second position – Holding the Balloon (see pp. 34-35), for five minutes.

Fourth, do the third Ba Duan Jin exercise: Holding Up a Single Hand Regulates the Spleen and Stomach (see pp. 70-71).

If you feel you need something even more powerful to deal with your hangover, try this. Boil some water. When it comes to the boil, put in some slices of fresh root ginger and let them boil in the water for two minutes. Then let the ginger water cool down. Add some honey for sweetness and drink the mixture slowly. Then swing your arms up and back round in gentle circles 30 to 50 times, stand in the second Zhan Zhuang position for five minutes, and finish off with the third Ba Duan Jin exercise (see pp. 70-71).

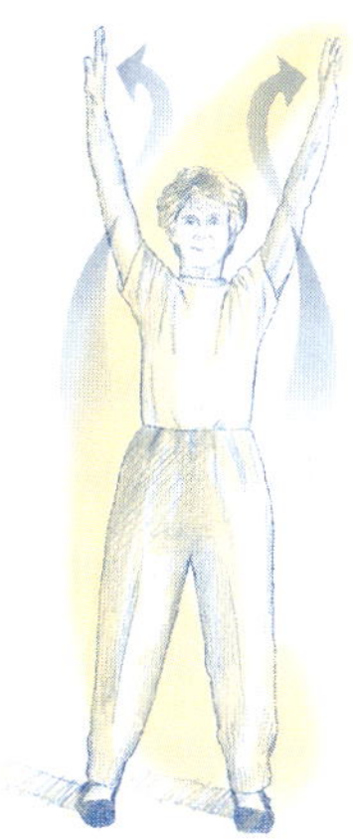

Warm up

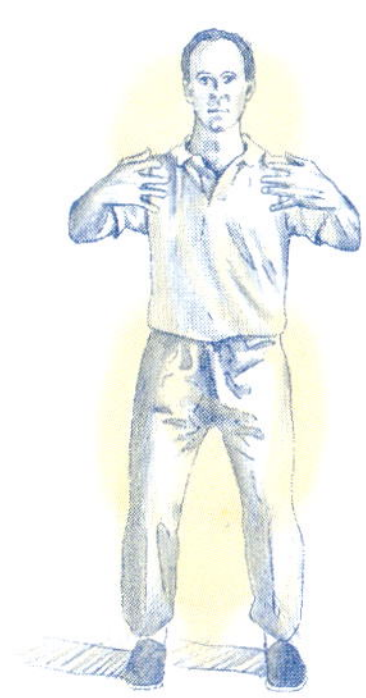

Holding the Balloon

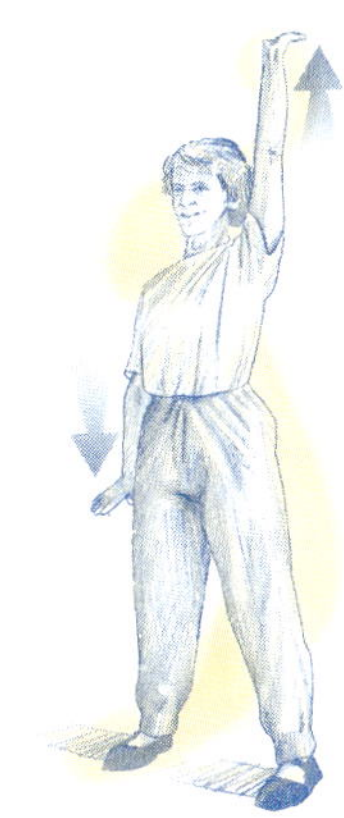

3rd Ba Duan Jin

TOOTHACHE

If you have toothache, the following will help relieve the pain. Stand in the second position – Holding the Balloon (see pp. 34-35), for two or three minutes. Keep your mouth gently closed with your tongue resting against the roof of your mouth. Saliva will form naturally. Imagine that the pain from your tooth is flowing away down your throat with the saliva.

For better results, dissolve a level teaspoon of salt in a glass of warm water. Use half the glassful to rinse your mouth thoroughly and spit out the water. The Chinese way is to drink the remaining water. After this, follow the procedure above. In most cases, the pain begins to subside within two or three minutes. Consult your dentist for treatment.

DEPRESSION

Anxiety, worry, listlessness, and depression are symptomatic of a serious imbalance in the energy of your nervous system. How can you help restore the natural balance?

If you feel so lacking in energy and motivation that you cannot even get out of bed, try Holding the Balloon in the lying position shown on page 167. Just doing that for 10 minutes (or for whatever length of time feels right for you) twice a day, will greatly calm your spirit and begin to revive your natural energy.

If you can go outside, stand while looking at the trees. Their energy is immensely beneficial. If you have an aquarium at home, gaze at the fish as they move and let your mind move with them. This can be of great help to compulsive worriers.

As your spirits begin to revive, adopt either the second position – Holding the Balloon (see pp. 34-35), or the third position – Holding your Belly (see pp. 84-85), and stand calmly for as long as you can manage. When you have reached your natural limit, lower your hands. Then rest the backs of your wrists on your lower back and do the eighth Ba Duan Jin exercise: Shaking the Body Wards Off all Illnesses (see p. 80). This is a powerful exercise for refreshing your internal organs and vibrating your spine. Your depression will lift as your Chi begins to circulate more vigorously.

INSOMNIA

If you have trouble sleeping, do the reclining Zhan Zhuang exercises in bed for as long as you can (see p. 167), then massage your abdomen (see "Relaxation before you sleep", p. 174). Some people may take an hour or so to calm down completely. After that almost everyone will sleep.

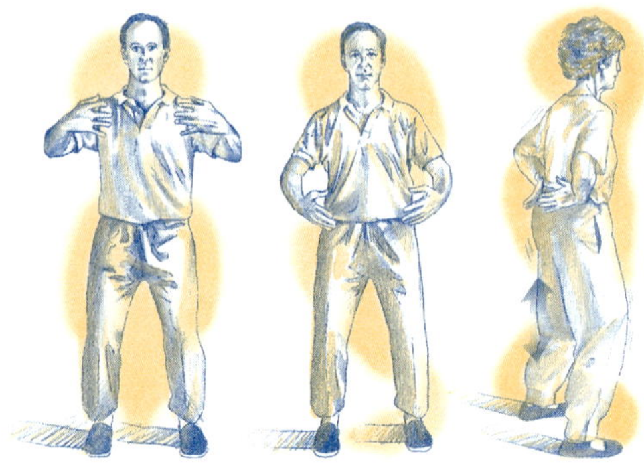

Holding your Balloon *Holding your Belly* *8th Ba Duan Jin*

MEDICAL BENEFITS

Enhanced blood circulation (see opposite) gives a positive stimulus to your central nervous system and brain. An experiment in Beijing, China, examined alertness. Those who were tested for their response to random, infrequent signals immediately after doing their normal Zhan Zhuang practice session had an average response time five times faster than the norm.

The calm and quiet mental state during the standing exercise has been shown to produce increasingly strong alpha waves within the brain, which indicate an alert but tranquil state. Zhan Zhuang exercise helps to eliminate exhaustion, headaches, dizziness, and nervousness.

Circulation

HIGH BLOOD PRESSURE

If you suffer from high blood pressure, try the following sequence of exercises every day. First, stand for two minutes in the third Zhan Zhuang position – Holding your Belly (see below, and pp. 84-85). As you stand in this position, imagine that you are outside in warm, gentle rain. This has a marvellous calming effect. Then do the third Ba Duan Jin exercise: Holding Up a Single Hand Regulates the Spleen and Stomach (see pp. 70-71). Finish with the fourth Ba Duan Jin exercise: Looking Back Like a Cow Gazing at the Moon (see pp. 72-73).

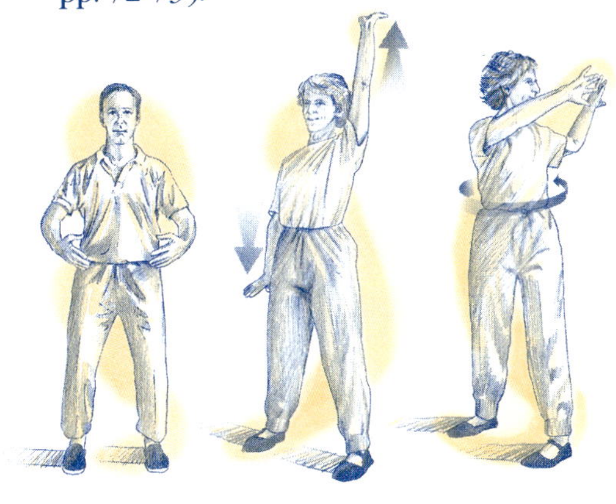

Holding your Belly *3rd Ba Duan Jin* *4th Ba Duan Jin*

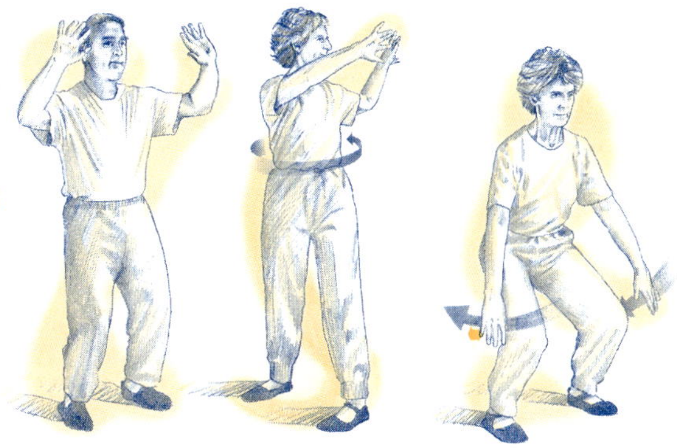

Balloon in Front of your Face *4th Ba Duan Jin* *6th Ba Duan Jin*

LOW BLOOD PRESSURE

If you have low blood pressure, follow this sequence. Start by holding the fifth Zhan Zhuang position: Holding the Balloon in Front of your Face (see pp. 92-93). Stay in that position for two or three minutes. Then do the fourth Ba Duan Jin exercise: Looking Back Like a Cow Gazing at the Moon (see pp. 72-73). Finish with the sixth Ba Duan Jin exercise: Touching the Feet with Both Hands Reinforces the Kidneys and Loins (see pp. 76-77).

Repeat this sequence of three positions once or twice a day.

MEDICAL BENEFITS

As you become calm and relaxed during Zhan Zhuang training, electrocardiograph measurements show that your heartbeat becomes slower and more powerful. The blood capillaries dilate, allowing a greater volume of blood to circulate through all the blood vessels.

An experiment conducted by Professor Yu Yong Nian at Teh Lu (Railway) Hospital in Beijing, measured blood counts of Zhan Zhuang practitioners before and after one hour of standing.

Haemoglobin levels had increased, as had the production of both white and red cells.

The protein within the red blood cells increased significantly, resulting in increased absorption of oxygen from the lungs by the blood, and improved circulation of the oxygen-rich blood to the rest of the body's internal organs.

Other studies have shown that Zhan Zhuang exercise lowers blood pressure in the majority of people. It has also helped people suffering from palpitations and heart murmur.

Skeletal problems

BACK PAIN

If you have a spinal disorder or a misalignment of your vertebrae that gives you back pain, you should seek special treatment. But if the cause of back pain is more simple, such as tension or fatigue, Zhan Zhuang exercises can help.

Stand for two or three minutes in the second Zhan Zhuang position – Holding the Balloon (see pp. 34-35). Then do an adaptation of the eighth Ba Duan Jin exercise, Shaking the Body Wards Off all Illnesses, as follows. Rise up on the balls of your feet; put the backs of your wrists into your lower back, just above your hips; gently arch your back and tilt your head back a little. Shake up and down on the balls of your feet and exhale in short bursts. Inhale smoothly, while still shaking. Complete 10 to 20 breaths, shaking all the time. This is a lovely massage for your whole spine.

ARTHRITIS

If you suffer from arthritis, first stand in the second Zhan Zhuang position – Holding the Balloon (see pp. 34-35) and follow this with the full eight Ba Duan Jin exercises every day. This will not cure your arthritis, for which special treatment is needed, but the exercises have been shown to arrest its further development.

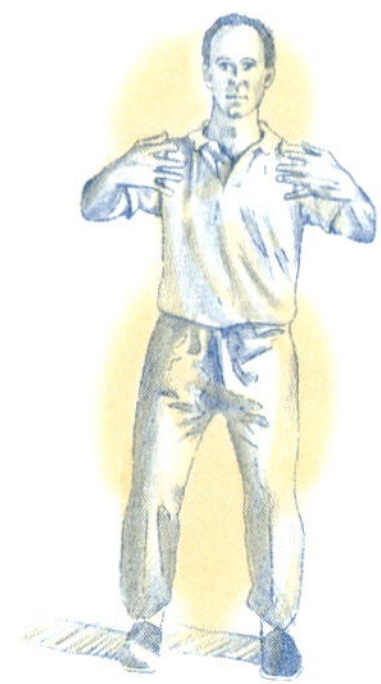

Holding the Balloon

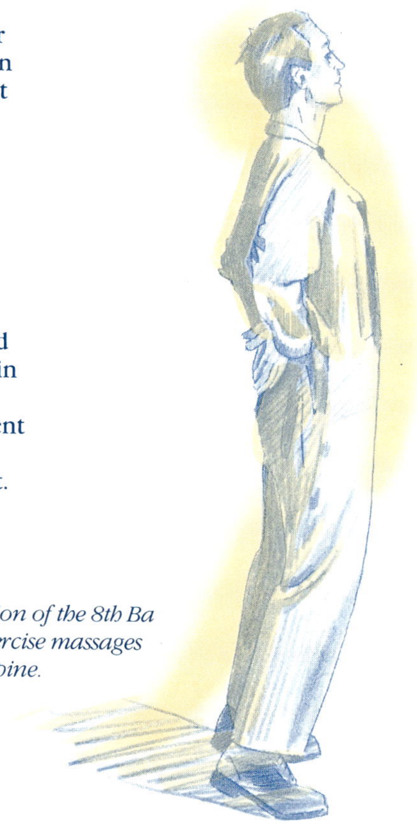

This adaptation of the 8th Ba Duan Jin exercise massages your whole spine.

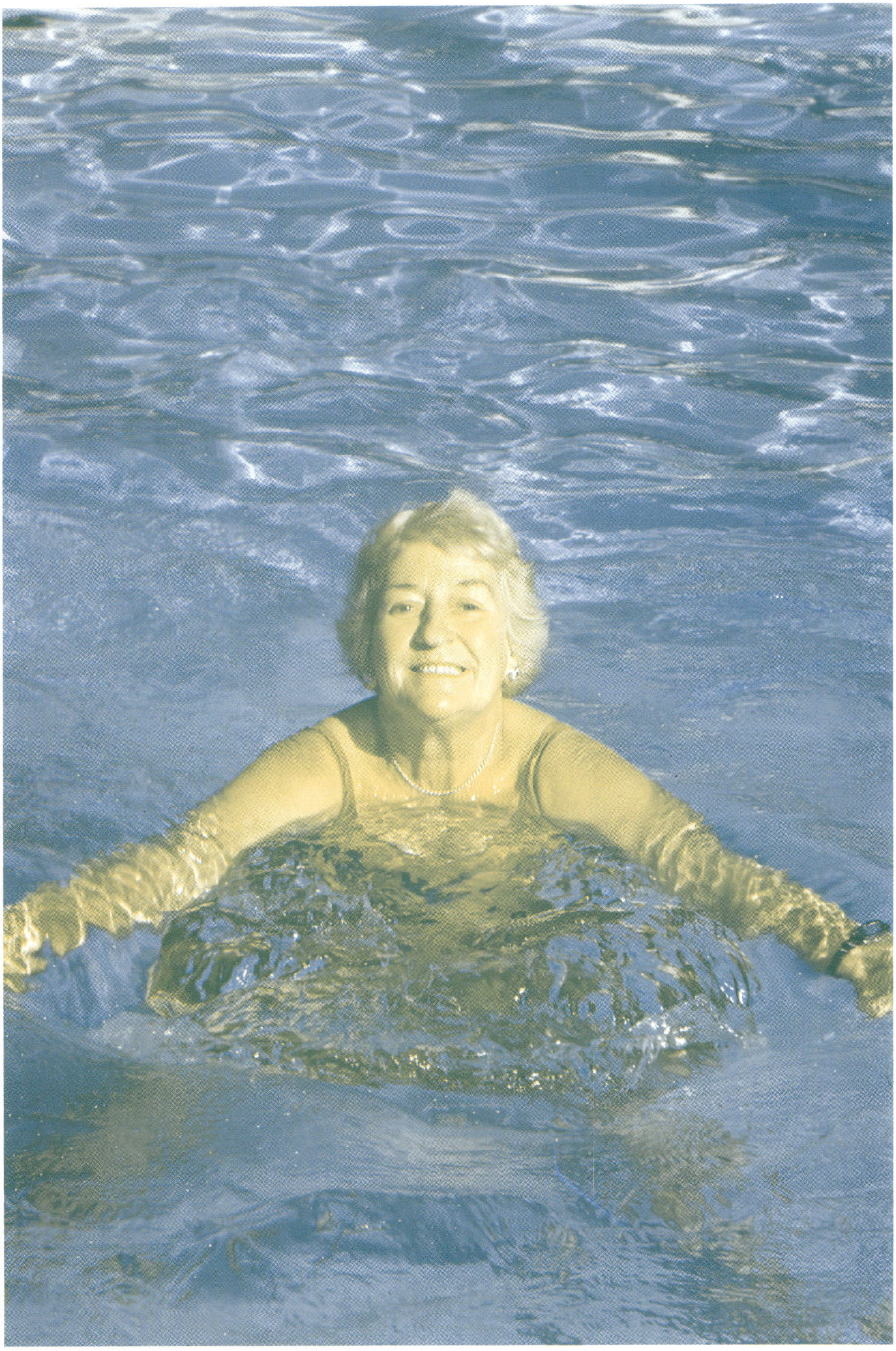

Returning to health

If you are in poor health or out of shape, or if you are a patient undergoing treatment, or recovering from an illness or an operation, you can adapt the Zhan Zhuang system to suit you. Each of these positions not only gives you support, but, in Chinese medical theory, gently increases the circulation of Chi in your body.

Caution: You should not attempt Zhan Zhuang without the advice of a competent instructor or your doctor, which you should follow in all cases.

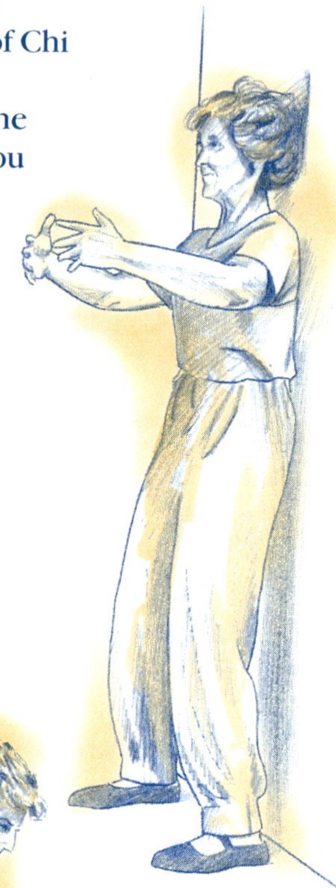

Lean against a wall for support.

STANDING

After a few minutes of warm up exercises, stand in either the first or second positions (pp. 28-29 and 34-35) for a maximum of 5 to 10 minutes. Do not force yourself to hold positions that cause you pain or exhaust you. If you cannot carry on, take a break. Try again the next day for a short period.

When you are standing, try leaning up against a wall. Put your back against the wall, bending your legs a little so that some of your weight is supported, and then try holding the balloon in the various positions (see right).

You can also try resting your hands on a table or on the back of a chair. Adopt the first position, breathe from the Tan Tien (see p. 42), then lean forward to rest your hands on the chair. Spread your weight equally over your hands and feet.

RAISING YOUR FOOT

If you have problems with your circulation and balance, you can try standing in any position with one foot raised and supported. For example, you can stand beside a chair and rest one foot on the seat of the chair. You can do this near a wall if necessary and use one hand to support yourself against the wall.

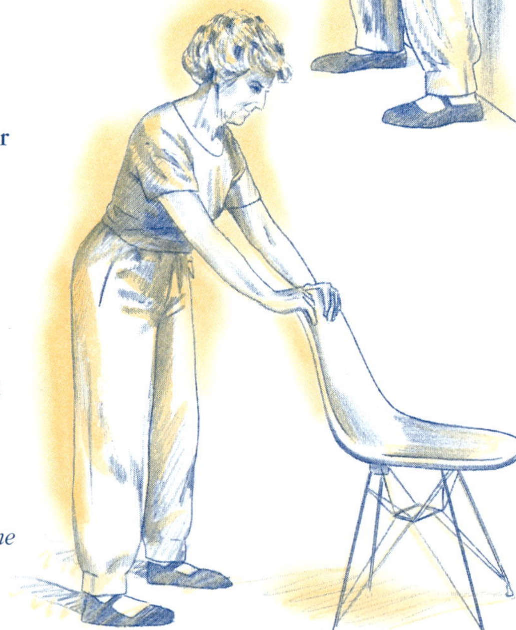

Let your hands take some of your weight.

SITTING

If you are weak and cannot stand, sit in a comfortable chair or on a sofa and place two beach balls under your arms (real beach balls, this time, not imaginary ones). The balls support your arms in the raised positions. You can also use the beach balls on a table top. Sit at the table and rest your arms on the two balls.

You can also practise with a beach ball under your feet while sitting (see right). This will take the strain off your legs, give your arms support, and reduce any strain on your abdomen. Try to lift your toes while resting only your heels on the ball.

LYING DOWN

If you are confined to bed or are extremely weak and can neither stand nor sit, you can practise Zhan Zhuang in a reclining position. For this, use the lying positions described on page 167 and the sleeping positions described in Chapter 8. Even if you are bedridden, the practice of Zhan Zhuang positions when lying down and sleeping can be of great benefit, since its effect is to build up and strengthen the centre of vital energy in your body (the Tan Tien). If the body's energy is recharged in this way, your return to health and vigour will be greatly assisted. It is wholly compatible with medical treatment.

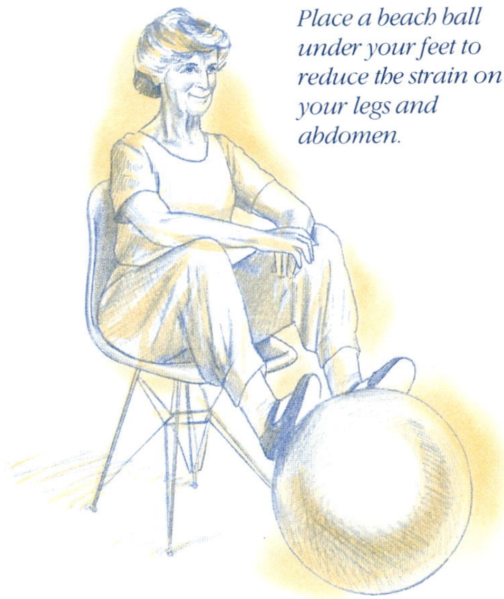

Place a beach ball under your feet to reduce the strain on your legs and abdomen.

Immunity and regeneration

Zhan Zhuang training increases the quantity and efficiency of the white blood cells, the body's defence against disease, improving its resistance to illness. Not only does Zhan Zhuang build up your body's defences against harmful external influences, it is also fundamentally regenerative. Because of the internal changes in your breathing rate, oxygen absorption, blood circulation, and digestive activity, your metabolic rate changes. Energy, rather than being consumed during exercise, is generated and stored.

First aid

Regular Zhan Zhuang practice improves the smooth flow of Chi inside you and so increases your ability to ease a sudden pain, or minor cut or burn, using the simple techniques outlined below. The more you have been able to release the blocked Chi within you through your practice, the more effective you will be in healing yourself and others. Seek medical advice for any serious conditions.

PAINS

If you or someone else has a sudden pain for any reason, such as toothache, the cause of the pain needs to be attended to. But you can help relieve the immediate pain by these three quick steps:

1. Rub your hands vigorously together for several seconds until they are warm;

2. Clap your hands together eight to ten times sharply and briskly;

3. Rest the palms of your hands firmly on the surface of your body above the point of the pain.

CUTS

If you or someone else has a cut, do the same as for pains (above), placing your palm very firmly over the cut and using your fingers to press your hand against the wound. Hold your hand in place for several minutes. The blood will clot naturally. Your Chi will speed the immediate healing process and, together with the spontaneous flow of blood from the wound, help resist infection.

BURNS

The Chinese first aid solution for minor burns is simple and available from your cupboard. Flood the burn with soy sauce. It works wonders.

Index

Bold type indicates main entry; *italics* indicate illustrations

A

aching, 55, 57
ageing, 168
ailments, self-treatment, 176
alcohol, 175
alertness, 182
aligning mind and body, 30–1
anger, 145
arms
  pain, 46
  tension, 49
arthritis, 26, 144
asthma, 177

B

Ba Duan Jin, 26, 63, **64–81**, 65, 167, 173–88
  exercises
  1. Supporting the Sky with Both Hands Regulates all Internal Organs, **66–7**
  2. Drawing a Bow to Each Side Resembles Shooting an Eagle, **68–9**
  3. Holding up a Single Hand Regulates the Spleen and Stomach, **70–1**
  4. Looking Back Like a Cow Gazing at the Moon, **72–3**
  5. Lowering the Head and Hips Removes Excess Heat from the Heart, **74–5**
  6. Touching the Feet with Both Hands Reinforces the Kidneys and Loins, **76–7**
  7. Clenching the Fists Increases Strength, **78–9**
  8. Shaking the Body Wards off all Illnesses, **80**
  for women, 164–7
  starting, 64, 65
back pain, 184
Balloon Fills with Water, 124
bicycling, 151
blood circulation, 20, 183
  increase, 55, 56
blood pressure, 171, 183
breathing, 42, 43
  abdominal, 42
  Tan Tien, 42, *42*
burns, 188

C

cardiovascular system, 78
central nervous system, 72
Chi, 18–19
  channels, 19, 20, 63
  flow, 98, 103
  network, 19
Chi Kung, 19
  ageing, 168
  applications, 20, 21
  research into, 53
  styles and schools, 21
childbirth, 164, 167
children, 160
Clenching the Fists Increases Strength, **78–9**
clothing, 26
common colds, 176
computer work, 148
constipation, 179
coughs, 176
cuts, 188

D

daily cycle of exercise, 142–3
daily exercise, 123
depression, 182
diet, 174, 175
digestion, 178–9
digestive system, 55, 174
do it yourself jobs, 152, 153
domestic work, 144–5
Drawing a Bow to Each Side Resembles Shooting an Eagle, **68–9**
  in pregnancy, 166
driving, 151

E

effects of Zhan Zhuang exercise, 51–2, 55–7
emotions, 175
endurance, 20, 88
energy
  circuit from tree, 134, 135
  in daily life, 141–57
  extending flow, 93, 103
  feeling the flow, 134–5
  from the galaxy, 136
  generation, 12, 16, 63
  of the human body, 18
  and movement, 141
  release of natural, 12, 16
  of the universe, 18
  wash, 145
Extending One Foot Forward (8th position), **114–15**, *115*

F G

facial muscles, 44
Feeling the Energy Flow, 134–5
feet, flow of Chi from, 78–9
fever prevention, 74
finger exercises, 148
first aid, 188
food, 174, 175
Full Circle, **96–7**
gall bladder, 70
gardening, 156
getting up, 142

H

hands, tension, 148
hangovers, 181
headaches, 162, 180
healing, natural process, 55
health, 11
  maintenance, 174–87
  returning to, 186–7
heart, 66, 68
  removal of excess heat, 74–5
heartbeat, 183
Holding the Ball on One Side (7th position), **112**, *112*
Holding the Balloon, (2nd position), 25, 26, **34–5**, *35*
  pain in arms, 46
  visualizing balloons, 35
Holding the Balloon in Front of your Face (5th position), **92–3**, *93*
Holding up a Single Hand Regulates the Spleen and Stomach, **70–1**
  in pregnancy, 166
Holding your Belly, (3rd position), 83, **84–5**
Hot Shower, Cold Shower, 125
housework, 144–5
hypertension, 72

I

imagery, 130
immune system, 20, 187
incense burning, 46, *47*
indigestion, 178
infants, 160
insomnia, 182
internal movement, 51–6
internal organs and systems, exercises for, 63
intestines, 66

K L

kidneys, 66, 72
knees, warm up exercises, 26, *26*
legs, tension, 47
leisure activities, 152–6
life cycle, 159–71
lifting heavy weights, 156–7
liver, 70
Looking Back Like a Cow Gazing at the Moon, **72–3**
Lowering the Head and Hips Removes Excess Heat from the Heart, **74–5**
lungs, 66, 68
lying position, 167, 187

M

menstruation, 39, 164
mental powers, 51
mental tension, 14, 41
mentality exercises, 41, 44–9, 124–36
meridians, 19, 63
middle age, 168–9

migraine, 180
mind, 19
  aligning with body, 30–1
  calming, 44–9
  increasing powers, 123–30
  moving from pain, 51
Mind in Action, 128
mind exercises
  Balloon Fills with Water, 124
  Hot Shower, Cold Shower, 125
  Moving Balloon, 126–7
  Pull of Magnets, 127
  Standing Near a Tree, 134
movement, 14, 19
  and energy, 141
Moving Balloon, 126–7
muscles, pain in, 51
  power, 16, 20
  relaxing, 41–9, 51
  tension, 51, 141
  tiring, 56

N O

narcotics, 175
nausea, 178
nervous system, 14, 41, 180–2
nervous tension, 19
numbness, 55, *57*
office work, 146–7
old age, 170

P

pain, back, 184
  first aid, 188
  moving mind from, 51, 52
  while exercising, 46, 49
period pain, 164, 165
posture, 19, 160
  pregnancy, 166
Pull of Magnets, 127
pulse rate, 51, 128

R

reading, 152
regeneration process, 55
relaxation, 14, 16, 41–9, 57, 130
  maintaining, 46–7
respiratory disorders, 176–7
Rising Up on One Leg (9th position), **118–19**, *119*

S

sensations, 52, 55–7
shaking, 56, *57*
  Shaking the Body Wards off all Illnesses, **80**
Shifting your Weight, 109
shopping, 144
shoulders, loosening, *27*
  tension, 49
sitting, 150, 152
  exercise during, 142
  office work, 146
skeletal problems, 184
skin, itching in old age, 170
sleeping positions, 143
smiling, 44
smoking, 162, 175
spleen, 70
sports, 154–5, 162
standing exercises, 25
  Full Circle, 96–7
  1st position, Wu Chi, 25, **28–9**, *38*, *64*, *97*
  2nd position, Holding the Balloon, *24*, 25, **34–5**, *97*
  3rd position, Holding your Belly, 83, **84–5**, *97*, *98*
  4th position, Standing in the Stream, 83, **88–9**, *97*, *99*
  5th position, Holding the Balloon in Front of your Face, **92–3**
  6th position, Weight on One Leg, **104–5**, 106, 107–8
  7th position, Holding the Balloon on One Side, **112**
  8th position, Extending One Foot Forward, **114–15**
  9th position, Rising Up on One Leg, *102*, **118–19**
  practice time, 29
  tension, 46
  whilst sleepy, 46
Standing in the Stream (4th position), **88–9**, *89*
  with sixth position, 106
stomach, 70
stress-related ailments, 162
Supporting the Sky with Both Hands Regulates all Internal Organs, *65*, **66–7**
  in pregnancy, 166
sweating, 51, 52, 55, 92

T U

Tai Chi Chuan, 26
Tan Tien, 31, *31*, 39, 42, *42*
  breathing, 42, *43*, 98
  focus of Chi network, 98
teenagers, 162
telephone calls, 146–7
television watching, 152
temper control, 162
temperature maintenance, 174
tension, 145, 174
  in hands, 148
  pain in arms and shoulders, 49
thigh muscles, 109
tingling sensation, 55, 63
toothache, 181, 188
Touching the Feet with Both Hands Reinforces the Kidneys and Loins, **76–7**
tranquillity, 130
travelling, 150–1
trees, energy, 31, 134
  growth, 103
trembling, 52, 56, 63, 92
universe, energy of, 18

W Y

walking, 151
Wang Xiang Zhai, 13, 17, 58–9, 135, 137
warm up routines, 25–6, 27
warmth, 57
Way of Energy, 14, 16, 153
weight control, 178
Weight on One Leg (6th position), **104–5**, *105*, *108*
  variations, 106, *107*
women, 164–5, 166–7
workplace, 146–9
Wu Chi, (1st position), **28–9**, *29*, *38*, *64*, *97*
Yang, 30
Yellow Emperor, 18
Yellow Emperor's Classic of Internal Medicine, 30
Yin, 30
Yu Yong Nian, Professor, 13, 52, 53, *54*, 58–9
  chart of, 55–6, *57*

Z

Zhan Zhuang, 11
  after childbirth, 167
  benefits, 11–21, 39, 55, 159
  daily exercise, 123
  exercises, 16
    1st position, Wu Chi, 25, **28–9**, *38*, *64*, *97*
    2nd position, Holding the Balloon, *24*, 25, **34–5**, 46, *97*
    3rd position, Holding your Belly, 83, **84–5**, *97*, *98*
    4th position, Standing in the Stream, 83, **88–9**, *97*, *99*
    5th position, Holding the Balloon in Front of your Face, **92–3**
    6th position, Weight on One Leg, **104–5**, 106, 107–8
    7th position, Holding the Ball on One Side, **112**
    8th position, Extending One Foot Forward, **114–15**
    9th position, Rising Up on One Leg, *102*, **118–19**
  medical benefits, 53, 55, 177, 179, 182, 183, 187
  menstrual effects, 164
  in middle age, 168–9
  in old age, 170
  in pregnancy, 166
  sensations during, 51–7
  sitting position, 142
  the system, 98, *99*
  for women, 164, 165, *165*, 166–7

Author's Acknowledgements

I am delighted to be able to introduce to a wide audience the art of Zhan Zhuang as developed by Grandmaster Wang Xiang Zhai. I have drawn extensively on his original manuscripts. Many teachers have made it possible for me to understand the art of internal strength. I am particularly grateful to Professor Yu Yong Nian for the wisdom he has shared with me and for his encouragement in the preparation of this book. I also owe much to my wife Villisa, and my three sons, Tin Yun, Tin Yu, and Tin Han – who have supported and inspired me. Nor would this edition have been possible without the untiring efforts of Richard Reoch and his partner Jane Ward.

My students have shown great patience in studying Zhan Zhuang despite the great leap of culture between East and West. Those who were models in this book include: Emma Davies; Beryl Heed; Andreas Michael; Jim McCarthy; Paul MacKay; Richard Reoch; Sean Stiles; Jane Ward, and Adrian White.

I would also like to express my appreciation to everyone at Gaia Books who has contributed to this project – to Imogen Bright, Joss Pearson, and Lucy Lidell who took the brave decision to publish a book on "standing still", to Eleanor Lines and Katherine Pate who worked meticulously and sensitively on the editing, and to Dave Thorp and Gail Langley who ensured a wonderful design.

Publisher's Acknowledgements

Gaia Books would like to thank: Susan Berry, Janine Christley, Eliza Dunlop, Lesley Gilbert, Jonathan Hilton, Libby Hoseason, Sarah Jarvis, Samantha Nunn, Sara Mathews, Dave Thorp, Susan Walby, and Mary Warren, for editorial and production work; Jill Halliday for the index; Simo Lam, Lam Tin Han, Lam Tin Yu, and Lam Tin Yun for modelling (see also author's acknowledgements); Gail Langley for the line drawings; Lucy Lidell for consultation; Studio 21 for the cover setting.

Photographic Credits

6–John Heseltine; 10–Science Photo Library; 15–Mark Jarvis Photo Library; 18–The Image Bank; 22–Mark Jarvis Photo Library; 24–Fausto Dorelli; 33–Mark Jarvis Photo Library; 37–Heather Angel; 38–Fausto Dorelli; 40–Tania Midgley; 45–Mark Jarvis Photo Library; 47–Fausto Dorelli; 48–Brian Rogers/Biofotos; 50–Mark Jarvis Photo Library; 54–Gaia Books; 60–Tania Midgley; 62, 82, 85–Fausto Dorelli; 87–Dave Thorp; 88–Fausto Dorelli; 91, 95–John Heseltine Photography; 100–The Image Bank; 102, 108–Fausto Dorelli; 111–Wildlife Matters; 113–Fausto Dorelli; 117, 121–Heather Angel; 122–Dave Thorp; 129–The Image Bank; 131–Andrew Lawson; 137–Image Bank; 138–Tania Midgley; 140–Mark Jarvis; 158–Bubbles Photo Library; 161–Fausto Dorelli; 163–Dave Thorp; 166–Bubbles Photo Library; 169–The Image Bank; 171–Bubbles Photo Library; 172–Fausto Dorelli; 185–The Image Bank.

Resources

Master Lam Kam Chuen gives Zhan Zhuang therapy, herbal and other treatments, for a range of disorders, at his clinic. He also teaches the Zhan Zhuang system.

The Lam Clinic
70 Shaftesbury Avenue
London W1V 7DF
Telephone: 0171 287 2114
or 0831 802 598
Fax: 0171 437 3118

Bibliography

There is very little in English on Zhan Zhuang. For background on this system read:

Reid, Howard, *The Book of Soft Martial Arts*, Gaia Books (UK), 1994 *The Way of Harmony*, Simon and Schuster (US), 1988

Wang Xuanjie, *Dachengquan*, Hai Feng Publishing Co Ltd, Hong Kong, 1988

The two great classics of Chinese culture on this subject are:

Lao Tzu *Tao Teh Ching*, (D. C. Lau English trans), Penguin (UK), 1963. (Gia-Fu Feng & Jane English trans), Random House (US), 1972.

Veith, Ilza (trans), *The Yellow Emperor's Classic of Internal Medicine*, University of California Press (US), 1972

Other books that cover aspects of Chi Kung and Chinese medical theory in English include:

Jiao Guorvi, *Qingong Essentials for Health Promotion*, China Reconstructs Press, China, 1988

Kaptchuk, Ted J., *Chinese Medicine: The Web that has no Weaver*, Century Hutchinson (UK), 1983

Maciocia, Giovanni, *The Foundations of Chinese Medicine*, Churchill Livingstone (UK and US), 1989

Scott, Julian, *Natural Medicine for Children*, Unwin Hyman (UK and Australia), Avon Books (US), 1990

Scott, Julian and Susan, *Natural Medicine for Women*, Gaia Books Ltd (UK), Avon Books (US), Simon & Schuster (Australia), 1991

Yang Jwing-Ming, *The Root of Chinese Chi Kung*, YMAA Chi Kung Series (US), 1989

Zhang Wingmu & Sun Xingyuan, *Chinese Qingong Therapy*, Shandong Science and Technology Press, China, 1985

ALSO PUBLISHED BY GAIA BOOKS

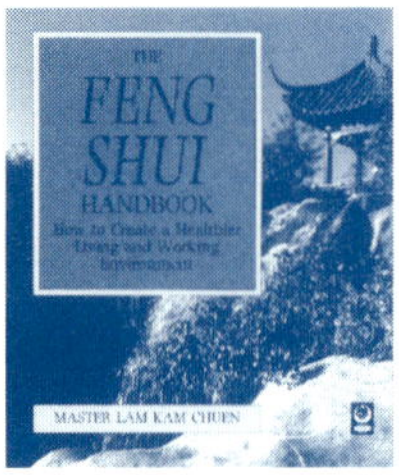

THE FENG SHUI HANDBOOK

Master Lam Kam Chuen

£12.99

ISBN 1 85675 047 7

Introduces the practical steps you can take to make your living and working environments healthier and more attuned to the life forces around you.

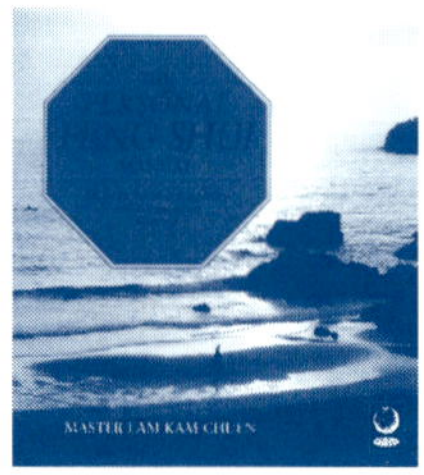

THE PERSONAL FENG SHUI MANUAL

Master Lam Kam Chuen

£12.99

ISBN 1 85675 053 1

Explains the basic principles of Feng Shui and gives step-by-step instructions on how to adjust your personal routine to promote health, wealth and happiness.

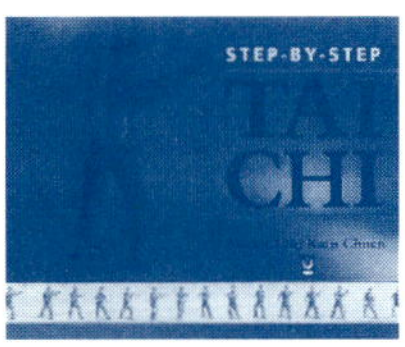

STEP-BY-STEP TAI CHI

Master Lam Kam Chuen

£11.99

ISBN 1 85675 066 3

Tai Chi exercises the body, soothes the mind and lifts the spirit. A guide for new and existing students of all Tai Chi styles.

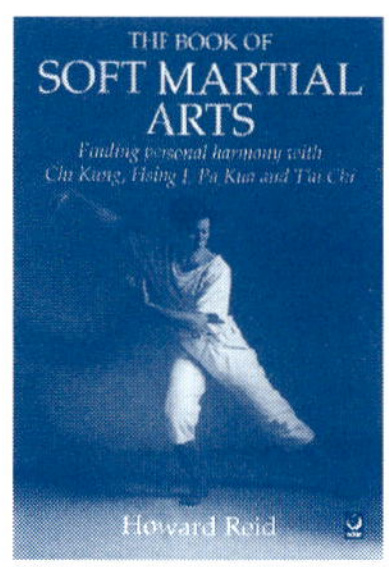

THE BOOK OF SOFT MARTIAL ARTS

Howard Reid

£11.99

ISBN 1 85675 096 5

A practical guide to classic Eastern exercises for cultivating inner strength and vital energy.

For a catalogue of titles published by Gaia Books, contact us by writing to Gaia Books, 20 High Street, Stroud, Gloucestershire, GL5 1AZ. T: 01453 752985 F: 01453 752987
e-mail info@gaiabooks.co.uk or visit our web site at http://www.gaiabooks.co.uk

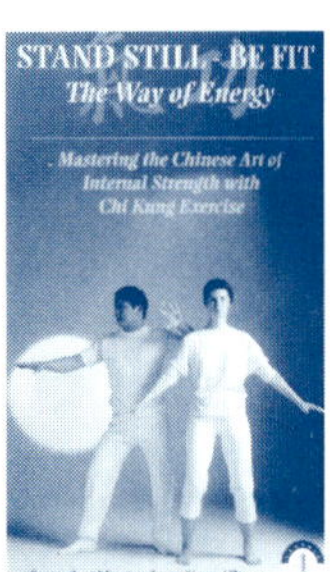

The video ***Stand Still - Be Fit*** contains the entire Channel 4 television series and it accompanies the book *The Way of Energy*. Using the ancient Zhan Zhuang system which requires little movement, Stand Still - Be Fit presents a step-by-step method that stimulates, massages, cleanses and revitalises the internal body, enhancing physical energy and improving your health and well being. The perfect fitness class for everybody of all ages to enjoy.

You can order ***Stand Still - Be Fit*** from Channel 4 Videos. Each copy costs £12.99 plus £1.50 for p & p. Please state how many copies you require and send cheques, made payable to Disc Distribution Ltd, Channel 4 Videos, PO Box 2640, London, W1A 3QU. Please allow 28 days for delivery.